Get the Pelvic Floor Back in Action

2nd Edition

A Physical Therapist's Insight into Rehabilitating Pelvic Dysfunction

Joanna Bilancieri, DPT
Author and Illustrator

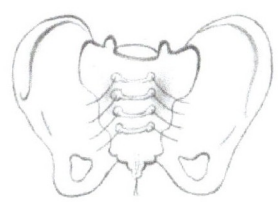

Editing Credits to Cynthia Farley

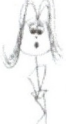 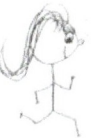

Copyright 2020

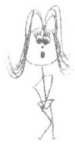

Thank You... Yes, You, My Patients!

To each and every patient who walked into my office, thank you. Thank you for the enlightening opportunity to work with you, to treat you, and to help you help yourself with your conditions. Without each and every one of you, this book would not be complete. Pelvic conditions are the lemons, but together we made, and continue to make, some amazing lemonade!

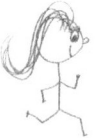

Table of Contents

- ❖ Prologue..8
- ❖ A Bit about Me, the Author............................9
- ❖ The Pelvic Floor's Functional
        Anatomy..14
    - Pelvic Floor Anatomy in
        Further Detail...15
    - Innervation of the Pelvic Floor.............18
    - An Overview of the Bladder and
        Its Innervation..20
    - An Overview of Common Pelvic
        Conditions..22

- ❖ Open Communication is Key to
        Rehabilitative Success..............................26

- ❖ The Almighty Kegel: Contraction
        of the Pelvic Floor....................................35
    - The Kegel's Resulting Neural
        Feedback..39

- ❖ The Gateway to Pelvic Floor
        Control Is the Isolation
        of Its Contraction....................................42
    - Helping Patients Find the
        Pelvic Floor Muscles..............................48
    - Building the Kegel Strength from
        Zero to Hero...51

❖ When Verbal and External Tactile Cues Are Not Enough, Give Biofeedback and Electrical Vaginal Stimulation a Try...................56
  • The Electrode and Electrical Stimulation..58
  • Electrical Stimulation in a Bit More Detail.....................................59
  • Electrical Stimulation Can Awaken the Pelvic Floor...61
  • A Few Similarities and a Few Differences between Electrical Stimulation and Biofeedback..............62

❖ Muscle Fiber Configurations Can Dictate Ease of Contraction, and the Lack Thereof...64
  • Asymmetries Often Underlie a Mechanical Disadvantage of the Pelvic Floor..68
  • Treating Pelvic Asymmetries....................77

❖ The Importance of a Home Exercise Program (...For Starters).......................79

❖ Stress Urinary Incontinence......................81
  • Stress Urinary Incontinence
  • Rehabilitation is Not 'Just Kegeling'.........87
  • Too Much Too Fast is NOT Recommended...95
  • Acquiring a Resting Tone in the Pelvic Floor Muscles..96

3

- Patients with Stress Urinary Incontinence Trudged into My Care, but with Rehabilitation, They Danced Out..98
- Tackling Stress Urinary Incontinence in a Bit More Detail..............................110
- Weakened Abdominal Musculature and a Tie to Stress Urinary Incontinence...120
- Stress Urinary Incontinence that Occurs Only with Exercise?..................121

❖ Urinary Urgency and Frequency.............128
- Key in the Door Syndrome........................130
- Artificially Induced Urinary Urgency... As a Treatment??...................................136
- Timed Voiding to Counter Urinary Urgency and Frequency........................138
- When Well-Timed, Isolated Kegels and Timed Voids Are Not Enough, Electrical Stimulation to the Rescue!...141
- Urinary Urgency Treatment Alternatives..142
- Mental Stress as a Culprit of Urinary Urgency and Frequency........................143
- Cortisol: Mental Stress's Link to Incontinence with Exercise?.................146
- Chemical Stimulants Can Create an Angry Bladder......................................151
- Nocturia: Nightly Urinary Frequency....................154

❖ Incomplete Voiding......................................156

- Electrical Stimulation Revisited,
    At a Higher Frequency............................163

❖ Mixed Incontinence and the
    Association of Incomplete Voids......164
  - Pelvic Floor Relaxation as
    Rehabilitation's Driving Force................165
  - A Complicated Case of
    Incontinence with Running....................174

❖ Pregnancy and Incontinence..................181

❖ Childbirth and Incontinence..................185

❖ Two to Four Weeks into
    Rehabilitation and a
    Regression Rears??............................188

❖ Space Invaders...
    (Prolapses, the " 'Celes")......................191

❖ Abdominal Exercise and
    Overcoming Incontinence....................195

❖ Abdominal Exercise and Prolapse..........198

❖ Pelvic Pain...200
  - Dyspareunia....................................215
  - Dyspareunia, Cases in Point..............219
  - Dyspareunia with Pain in Flux............223
  - A Sneak Attack on Dyspareunia...........224
  - A Handful of Conditions

> Associated with Pelvic Pain:
> Endometriosis, Interstitial Cystitis,
> Tumors, Calcified Masses, and
> Uterine Fibroids..................................229

❖ The Role of the Core in
    Fighting Pelvic Pain............................237

❖ Nutrition, a Pelvic Pain Fighter..............239
- Nutrition's Fight Against Pain
  in a Bit More Detail...........................241
- Nutrients that Flush Retained Fluid
  May Increase Bladder Irritation.........242
- Turmeric:
  A Natural Anti-Inflammatory............244

❖ The Power of the Healing Touch:
    Diagnostic and Therapeutic.................246
- Every Little Bit of Pain Relief Helps......254
- A Team Approach...............................256

❖ Pain with Emotional Stress is NOT
    Psychosomatic.......................................258

❖ A Few More Words on Sexual
    Trauma..266
- Overcoming Emotional Stress as a
  Sexual Abuse Survivor:
  Step Outside Yourself to
  Treat Yourself....................................267
- In Overcoming Anguish of a
  Trauma, Sometimes Forgiveness
  Is Not the Answer..............................270

- ❖ A Few Words Specifically for Men..........272
- ❖ Disorders Involving Control of the Pelvic Floor, without a Drop of Incontinence........................273
- ❖ In Conclusion..................................278
- ❖ Epilogue..280
- ❖ References....................................281
- ❖ Index...289

Disclaimer

The author, illustrator, editor, printer, formatter, and publisher of this book recommend seeking medical attention for medical advice. The contents of this book do not substitute for the medical attention and the needs addressed by individuals' clinicians. The author, illustrator, editor, formatter, printer, and publisher of this book intend to present correct information at the time of press. Any and all information utilized is at the reader's own risk. If any techniques, exercises, treatments, instructions, and/or other materials are utilized, the reader does so at his or her own will and risk. Any performance or use of the techniques, exercises, treatments, instructions, and/or other materials is at the reader's own will and risk and should not be performed or utilized if any harm or pain develops or worsens. The author, illustrator, editor, printer, formatter, and publisher of this book do not assume and do disclaim liability for any errors or damages resulting from any cause.

Prologue

"Hello! I was wondering if you treat patients with pelvic pain. I have endometriosis…"

Amidst writing this book, I received a phone call from a woman with a timid, yet hopeful voice. This sweet voice so very politely asked if I treated patients with pelvic pain, particularly those with endometriosis. I responded with a calm, drawn out, yet emphatic, "Yyyesss." My tone and answer induced a smiling sigh of relief and a welling tear on the other end of the line. The woman's voice resonated with hope, as if a long arduous journey had ended, and she was ready to venture through the proverbial tunnel with a beaming light calling her name. We talked about the ways we could together tackle her condition and we set an appointment to meet. Upon hanging up the telephone, I smiled. Tears of fulfilling joy rolled down my cheek. Those very words fueled my fire to continue to decipher the complexities of pelvic disorders and to help lead patients down the road to recovery.

A Bit about Me, the Author

I would like to take you on a journey healing several debilitating conditions that involve the pelvic region. My strategies incorporate research as well as cases I have seen from 2001 to the present. Men have pelvic floor disorders, such as urinary incontinence and pelvic pain, and do indeed greatly benefit from pelvic floor rehabilitation. However, the number of women I have treated is by far greater than the number of men. Therefore, the cases I present on this journey are women who have overcome or managed a myriad of conditions of pelvic dysfunction.

As a college undergraduate I was fortunate to attend Yale University, focusing my attention on pre-medical biology with an emphasis in physiological psychology. I also delved into anthropology and history. My coursework intertwined bodily systems with cultural and artful underlays and ignited my appreciation for all of life's functions. I left Yale understanding that even the most minute details are integral segments of the art form we call a human being.

While studying for my Doctorate of Physical Therapy at the University of Southern California, one of my research projects targeted the evaluation and treatment of urinary incontinence, even though incontinence was *not* embedded in USC's curricula. After my group's presentation, however, my professors informed me that they would see to it that incontinence was indeed added to the curricula in the ensuing years.

Having just graduated and excited to start my career as a physical, or physio-, therapist, a serendipitous opportunity arose to work side by side with a brilliant, world-renowned urogynecologist and obstetrician by the name of Dr. Cynthia Mosbrucker. I was fortunate to witness her surgeries and to treat mutual patients. In 2007, I established my own boutique-style practice, small and individualized, and continued to benefit from the interactions with my urogynecologist/obstetrician friend. To this day, we continue to work as a team, as I do with many clinicians in rehabilitating pelvic dysfunction. Together, we strive to succeed at conquering pelvic conditions.

Over the years, I have encountered remarkable cases of pelvic dysfunction that required thinking inside, outside, and all around the proverbial box. Cases such as stress urinary incontinence, urinary urgency and frequency, incomplete voiding, pelvic pain, scoliosis, back pain, neuritis, sacroiliac dysfunction, endometriosis, interstitial cystitis, painful intercourse, and persons with any combination of these conditions have walked into my care. My intent as the author of this book is to share my clinical findings and gathered opinions. When the question 'why' is left unanswered by my literature searches, I share my own speculations. As of the completion of this piece, I had not found literature to support *all* of my findings. Furthermore, my intent is not to inundate my audience with a plethora of research articles. My findings left unsupported by literature are open for discussion. I hope to spawn interest in my readers to continue the search for the many possible answers to the question 'why', to perform individual research, and to report back! Medical science is a team effort, and with a team, more questions can be answered and more cases can be treated successfully.

I welcome audiences of all backgrounds: Patients, clinicians, folks concerned about partners, friends and family members of those with pelvic dysfunction, and folks looking to minimize the chance of becoming a patient.

What is My Specialty?
People. I Specialize in People.

Although pelvic rehabilitation is considered a 'specialty', I do not find it appealing to be considered a 'specialist' in any one type of therapy. In my opinion, in order to adequately treat, a view of the whole person is paramount. Only when we see how all the bodily systems interconnect can we fully rehabilitate. Thus, to the ever-present question, "What is my specialty?" I respond, "People. I specialize in *people*."

Acquiring a solid background in physical, or physio-, therapy lays the groundwork for rehabilitating pelvic dysfunction. Such knowledge includes the mindfulness that the whole body is connected in one way or another. Orthopedic, neurological, and psychological conditions may all seep into the pelvic region and contribute to pelvic disorders. Considering all systems is imperative to unlocking the rehabilitative code.

Numerous conditions revolve around inadequate control of the pelvic floor musculature. Some conditions are straightforward and uncomplicated. Oftentimes, however, multiple conditions weave together into a loom that requires intricate thought and dissection. Singly, one impairment may not have too detrimental of an effect on a patient's function. However, adding one impairment to another may create a scenario such as that of the proverbial straw. In cases of pelvic dysfunction, each straw must be discovered and conquered to get patients on the mend and back in action!

It is essential to tackle disorders involving the pelvic floor with a holistic approach and a constant investigation of all of the bodily systems and their interactions. The evaluation should be an ongoing process that extrapolates pieces of a puzzle and untangles any and all of the causes of a condition. With an ongoing query of causes and effects, each treatment technique should be applied with careful concern for optimal and efficient results. All the strategic treatment techniques can then morph into a masterpiece entitled, 'Pelvic Dysfunction Rehabilitation'.

Now Let's Get To It...

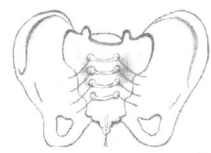

The Pelvic Floor's Functional Anatomy

The pelvic floor is an interactive network of musculature, ligaments, and supportive fascia. Its constituent muscles can contract and relax to allow for controlled urination and defecation, support of the organs of the pelvic cavity, and support of the spinal segments and pelvic joints. Strung from one region of the pelvis to another, the muscles of the pelvic floor attach to bony structures and soft connective tissues of the perineal region. Some of the muscles are directly controlled by a voluntary contraction. Others, in normalcy, contract automatically.[1] A balance of contraction time and relaxation time can allow for adequate muscle tone and comfort.

The pelvic floor is divided into multiple layers. The layer often referenced in medical diagnoses is the innermost layer, known as the pelvic diaphragm.[1] Medical diagnoses of pelvic floor weakness and spasm often point to the levator ani, one of the pelvic diaphragm's fundamental muscles.

The pelvic floor as a whole extends from the coccyx (tailbone) and ischial spine, which is situated at the posterior aspect of the pelvis. The anterior-most fibers anchor onto the pubis (pubic bone), which is situated at the anterior, inferior aspect of the pelvis, and the connective tissues therearound. Small branches of muscle attach to the urethra, clitoris, vagina, and anus. Altogether, the pelvic floor muscles appear to form a figure eight around the anus and collectively around the vagina and urethra. Such a design enables their contractile abilities to close each orifice, act as a supportive harness for the pelvic organs,[1] and keep the joints of the spine and pelvis stable.

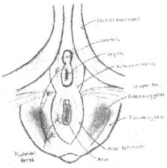

Pelvic Floor Anatomy in Further Detail

In anatomic detail, the multiple layers of pelvic floor musculature can be further broken into muscle segments and their constituent muscle fibers. Anatomists differ in their opinions of the names for each muscle segment, the separation of each segment, and the actual number of muscle layers within the pelvic floor.[1] My aim is to provide a simple overview of the anatomy to help you understand the pelvic floor's inner workings for rehabilitation.

The outer layer of the pelvic floor consists of the bulbocavernosus and ischiocavernosus muscles anteriorly, and the external anal sphincter posteriorly. The bulbocavernosus runs centrally, whereas the ischiocavernosus spans diagonally and laterally. With the bulbocavernosus circling the vagina and urethra, and the external anal sphincter circling the anus, the two appear to form the aforementioned figure eight.[1] Making fists with our hands side by side can simulate a visual of the outer muscle layer's contractions on a larger scale.

    As previously mentioned, the inner layer of the pelvic floor, known as the pelvic diaphragm, houses the levator ani muscle. The inner layer also contains the coccygeus muscle and the connective tissue known as the arcus tendineus. The coccygeus sits in the posterior aspect of the pelvic floor attaching to the coccyx (tailbone), the sacral spine, and the ischium of the pelvis. The arcus tendineus spans from the pubis (pubic bone) anteriorly to the inferior portion of the pelvis posteriorly.[1] The pelvic floor's anatomy is clearly quite intricate. But, to describe the levator ani muscle, we shall get into *epic* detail…

    The levator ani itself consists of the pubococcygeal muscle fibers medially and the iliococcygeal muscle fibers laterally. The pubococcygeus spans from the pubis (pubic bone) to the coccyx (tailbone), and is therefore aptly named. The pubococcygeus has smaller subsets of muscle fibers that attach to the rectum, anus, vagina, and urethra. These muscles are fitly named with their origin and attachment sites. The iliococcygeus originates toward the posterior aspect of the pelvic floor at the arcus tendineus. The iliococcygeus spans to the posterior, inferior portion of the pelvis, latching onto the ischial spine and coccyx (tailbone). These muscles weave together to create the levator plate, which supports the pelvic organs and contracts to deliver continence.[1] (See Figure 1.)

Figure 1. Pelvic floor musculature.

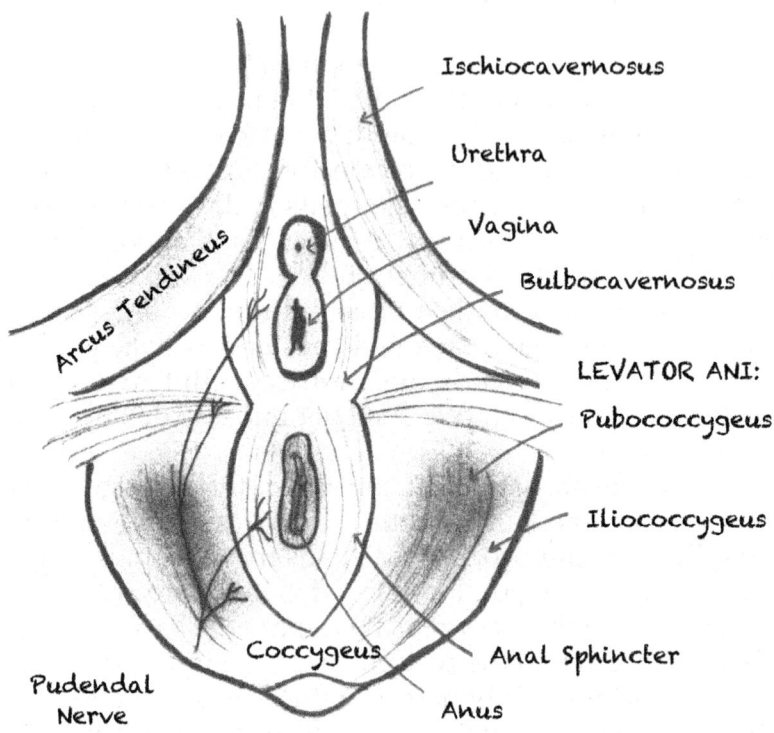

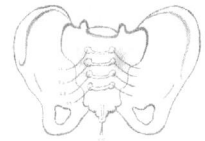

Innervation of the Pelvic Floor

The pelvic floor muscles receive their nerve supply from the pudendal nerve, which is comprised of sacral nerves S2-S4[2] and the anterior branch of sacral nerve S5.[1,3] (See Figure 2.) Damage to the pudendal nerve or to any of its constituents, especially S3-S5, may be linked to incontinence,[3] the loss of urinary and/or fecal control. Sacral nerve S3 has been shown to have a particularly strong connection to urinary continence[3] (urinary control), thus damage to S3 may contribute to a lack thereof. Disrupting these nerves, as with a herniated disc, with ilial (pelvic) asymmetry, and/or with muscular compression, can compromise the ability to adequately contract and relax the pelvic floor muscles, as I have seen in several of my patients. If pelvic dysfunction stems from an impaired nerve, the underlying cause of neural impairment should be addressed along with pelvic floor muscle training. Pelvic floor muscle training, which will be discussed in detail in later sections, including *'Building the Kegel Strength from Zero to Hero'*, should include improving contractile ease and/or contractile release, as when re-establishing muscle control in a lower extremity after sciatic nerve damage. Muscle conditioning may only be effective, though, if the nerve feeding into the muscle is returned to health. If damage to the pudendal nerve or its constituents is present, rehabilitation of the pelvic floor's overall control may only be *fully* addressed if the neural integrity is restored.

Figure 2. Innervation of the pelvic floor.

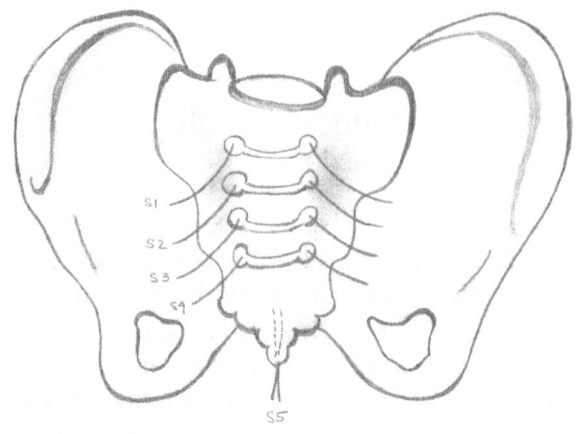

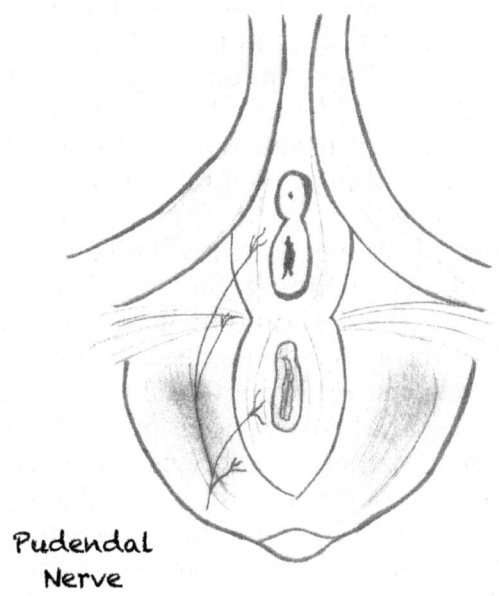

Pudendal Nerve

19

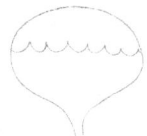

An Overview of the Bladder and Its Innervation

The bladder houses the detrusor muscle, which can contract in response to being stretched by rising amounts of urine. There is an internal sphincter that resides at the inferior aspect of the bladder at the bladder's opening to the urethra. The detrusor muscle and internal sphincter are innervated by the autonomic nervous system, the portion of the central nervous system in charge of the 'fight or flight' response and its counterpart to calm.[2]

Under normal circumstances, as urine trickles into an empty bladder, the internal sphincter reflexively shuts, and filling of the bladder ensues. The nerves that detect the commencement of bladder filling and reflexively close the internal sphincter are derived from thoracic and lumbar nerves T10-L2. These nerves converge to form the hypogastric and pelvic nerves and are sympathetic in nature (as are those that are responsible for the 'fight or flight' response). The bladder normally does not contract before it is at least half full. The hypogastric and pelvic nerves ordinarily signal to keep the internal sphincter closed as the bladder fills to half way, keeping urine from passing through to the urethra.[4]

Once the bladder's urine level rises above the halfway point and the bladder is approaching full capacity, the stretch placed on the bladder's detrusor muscle usually provokes the detrusor to contract, and an urge to void develops. Voiding can then proceed as the internal sphincter opens and urine flows through the urethra. The nerves that are responsible for contracting the bladder's detrusor muscle and opening the internal sphincter are parasympathetic (calming) in nature and stem from sacral nerves S2-S4. Should urinating not be appropriate or desired, despite the bladder being beyond half full, pelvic floor muscle contraction can normally close the external sphincter and counter the bladder's contraction. Should voiding be appropriate, the pelvic floor muscles can ordinarily relax to open the external sphincter and allow the void to ensue.[4]

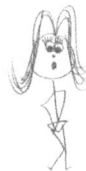

An Overview of Common Pelvic Conditions

In 1948, a gynecologist by the name of Dr. Arnold Kegel was onto something monumental. Dr. Kegel published the first accounts of the pelvic floor's muscular contractions and their effect on pelvic floor control. He described inadequate pelvic floor contraction as "genital relaxation".[5] The contraction of the muscles surrounding the genitals was thusly named a 'Kegel'. Determining the value of a Kegel was an epic breakthrough in rehabilitation. The Kegel continues to be instrumental in rehabilitating numerous conditions that, if left untreated, could render a life of pain, frustration, and limitation.

Not only do several women suffer from pelvic floor weakness and from the inability to control the contraction and relaxation of the pelvic floor muscles, many also lack the knowledge of *where to find* these muscles. Lack of pelvic floor muscle strength and control may stem from a myriad of confounding factors, including pelvic asymmetry and altered muscle fiber length, neural compromise, physical trauma, and mental anguish manifesting in physical tension. These factors and others will be analyzed in their own sections. Restoring control over the pelvic floor musculature can be a complicated process, but well worth every step for an immense population with a number of pelvic conditions.

The following common pelvic conditions have presented in my clinic and will be explored in their own sections:

***Stress urinary incontinence (SUI)** constitutes urinary leakage upon application of physical stress to the abdominal and/or pelvic cavity. Such physical stress can accompany activities such as lifting, sneezing, coughing, changing position, running, and jumping. The forceful application of pressure onto the bladder with these activities can render difficulty in keeping the external urinary sphincter closed, and uncontrolled voiding can ensue.

***Urinary urgency or urge incontinence** is a premature need to urinate, in which a small amount of urine can trigger a strong, uncontrollable urge. This strong urge may lead to uncontrolled urination even if minimal urine has trickled into the bladder.

***Urinary frequency** can accompany urinary urgency, as it constitutes a *need* to urinate *more frequently* than the bladder fills beyond its halfway point.

***Incomplete void** is the entrapment of urine in the bladder despite having just attempted to empty the bladder's contents. Incomplete void may associate with a difficulty in fully relaxing the pelvic floor muscles. It may also stem from premature contraction of the pelvic floor muscles, which halts the urine stream before the bladder has fully emptied.

***Pelvic pain** may stem from a number of conditions including pelvic joint asymmetry, trauma, scoliosis, muscle imbalance, muscle weakness, muscle guarding, and the presence of calcified masses, cysts, fibroids, and/or scar tissues. Pelvic pain may also stem from a combination of any of these entities plus others. Pelvic pain may involve inadequate control over the pelvic floor muscles. A patient may have enough control to secure continence, but not quite enough to support the torso or to allow for full relaxation. Pelvic pain can accompany inflammation, as with *interstitial cystitis,* and tissue overgrowth, as with *endometriosis* and *fibroids.* Aside from rendering pain, bouts of inflammation and extraneous tissue growth may also complicate the control of the pelvic floor musculature. (*Endometriosis, interstitial cystitis (IC),* and *fibroids* are further discussed in the section entitled '*Pelvic Pain*'.)

***Prolapses** are occurrences of space invasion whereby pressure is applied to a vaginal wall causing the wall to protrude. The bladder, uterus, urethra, rectum, small bowel,[6,7] and the vagina itself[6] can all essentially *fall* into the vaginal walls.[6,7] The prolapses can invoke pain and incontinence in addition to creating problems in their organs of derivation.

Disorders with a less than straightforward cause include those involving mental and emotional stress harnessed in the pelvic region. Such stress can create painfully tense and guarded muscles, and may interfere with pelvic floor muscle control. These cases may be as simple to treat as lending an ear to allow a patient to unload her stress. They may also be as difficult as helping a patient work through anguish that sets her emotions into a tailspin, while also treating her impairments precipitated by a frightening physical trauma. A survivor of sexual assault exemplifies such a case.

Whether pelvic conditions are simple or complicated, common or rare, control over the pelvic floor musculature can be paramount to recovery. Gathering the details of the conditions, addressing their underlying causes, and helping a patient gain control over the involved musculature are areas where physical therapists can strut their stuff.

Onto Rehabilitation...

Open Communication is Key to Rehabilitative Success

Achieving control over pelvic conditions should start with one rehabilitative element: Open communication between the clinician and the patient. There is not just *one* means to solve pelvic dysfunction, but all of the solutions should share the key ingredient of open communication. Open communication can stem from the clinician's sincere concern for the patient's condition and the patient's ability to disclose personal information. For many with pelvic dysfunction, the causes and effects of their conditions can be challenging to discuss. Such challenges may stem from embarrassment in discussing a private region of the body, from difficulty in rehashing a trauma, or from a feeling of shame, particularly if the patient has a history of sexual abuse. The clinician's open mind and welcoming ear can create a setting in which the patient finds ease in communicating. Listening wholeheartedly can give the patient confidence that she will not be judged and can encourage the flow of communication to help the healing process begin.

Treatment should begin with listening to understand, not just to respond. Good listeners listen with ears *and eyes*, taking the time to digest the spoken words, the emotional tones, and the body language. A patient's body language can be even louder than her spoken words.

Listening is waiting until the patient not only finishes a sentence, but also finishes a thought. Instead of quickly jumping to the next question, a good listener gives time for silence. That momentary silence can brew the next words that leave a patient's mouth. Oftentimes those words are just what the clinician was seeking. Further questioning can take place, but in due time.

Allowing a patient to divulge information at her own pace can help to give her power over her condition. Setting this pace can build a patient's confidence in handling her condition, which often involves the frustrating loss of a bodily function. Some patients have no problem talking about their conditions. Some say they have been trying to get a grasp of their incontinence or pelvic pain for so long, they no longer feel any embarrassment. Others feel as though they have been to so many clinicians they no longer find any difficulty talking about their conditions. Still others have difficulty not only finding the words to explain their symptoms, they also have difficulty disclosing from where their problems arise. Regardless of the situation, listening true to form can encourage the patient to communicate her story. And, the greater the amount of information shared by the patient the more tools the clinician has to help her heal.

To assist patients in divulging their stories, I have found that it helps to make it known that they are not alone, rather they are among an immense number of people with pelvic conditions. To my clinician readers, be prepared to have examples of cases to share. Enlightening a patient that she is among many people with similar conditions can ease her tension. Be careful, though, not to clump all patients with pelvic disorders together. Make sure each patient understands that although she is among many with a pelvic condition, she is an individual who will be treated as such, and that together you will find her individual recipe for recovery!

A clinician's line of questioning should pursue the details of the patient's history to further unveil culprits of pelvic conditions. Helpful questions inquire of a pain or dysfunction pattern and an association of pain or dysfunction with specific activities. The patient may note a particular time of day when symptoms are especially painful or when it is more difficult to accomplish daily tasks without urinary leakage. The line of questioning should disclose the causes of pelvic dysfunction, such as childbirth, trauma, neglect of the pelvic floor muscles, and stress, while exposing the patient's level of pelvic floor control, or lack thereof.

A written questionnaire is a useful tool for a clinician to start an evaluation. (See Figure 3.) The written questionnaire allows a clinician to retrieve several pieces of general, yet pertinent, information with time efficiency. Having a patient read the questions and write her answers is a faster means of attaining such information than verbally questioning the patient. A verbal discussion can then draw from the answers on the written questionnaire to disclose specific patient details.

There are numerous orthopedic, neurologic, and other types of medical conditions that can interfere with pelvic floor muscle alignment, trigger pelvic pain, and/or affect healing rates. The questionnaire presented in Figure 4 is a useful tool for patients to reveal such medical information. Pain levels and patterns, histories of surgeries and comorbidities, and medications that are currently taken are all important factors to consider when diagnosing and treating. Concurrent medical conditions may interfere with the pelvic condition's rehabilitation process and may contribute to the dysfunction's cause.

The questionnaires not only offer efficient assistance in evaluating and diagnosing pelvic floor conditions, they go one step further. For the patients who find it embarrassing to *speak* of the causes and details of their conditions, it may be easier to offer information in written form. This scenario is especially true for those who have endured sexual trauma and other forms of abuse. One of my patients actually thanked me for having a written questionnaire. She told me it allowed her to get the stress of a trauma figuratively off her chest, and, consequently, literally out of her pelvic cavity! The questionnaire acted, in a sense, as a therapeutic journal. Writing the answers on the questionnaire may ease the burden of verbally telling a painful story and can begin the treatment by alleviating at least some of the stress associated with the pelvic condition.

Verbal communication should continue throughout the course of successive treatment sessions to paint the complete picture of the conditions' causes and effects, and to determine the success of treatment strategies. Open communication can assist a clinician in knowing which treatment methods are effective and which are not, prompting the advancement of certain strategies and the withdrawal of others. Each day brings new scenarios to a patient's life. Through open communication, the patient and clinician can work together to determine which treatment methods are most beneficial to each scenario. By communicating the effects of activities on her condition or pain level, a patient can help her clinician determine the most appropriate means of restoring her ability to perform each activity without detriment.

By helping to guide treatments along the correct path, a patient can start to help herself recover and assume power over her condition. With a clear understanding of her impact on the recovery process, a patient can strongly believe she is not just the person afflicted with the condition, but is a key player on the rehabilitation team.

Dissecting myriads of idiosyncrasies for each condition can make rehabilitation an evolving process. It is important to not only understand the inner workings of the pelvic region, but to also understand how life's activities play into the dysfunction. This dissection can best be tackled with the patient and clinician acting as a team. This team effort can give the patient power over her condition as she assumes the responsibility of communicating her status. The patient's feedback can help the clinician decide which methods are best to help her claim victory over her pelvic conditions. Thus, strong communication can shine as a key ingredient in uncovering the sources of the conditions, and in moving the rehabilitative process in the direction that gets the patient back in action!

Figure 3: A questionnaire presented upon intake specifically targeting pelvic floor conditions.

Incontinence & Pelvic Pain History
Page 1

Name:
Age:
Date:

Please describe your condition:

Is there a particular experience or series of events associated with the onset of your condition?

Do you experience urinary leaking (incontinence)?
If yes, did it commence abruptly or gradually?

Do you experience pelvic pain?
If yes, did it commence abruptly or gradually?

Do you experience pain with intercourse?
If yes, did it commence abruptly or gradually?

Do you experience incontinence with any of the following activities:
Exercising?   Coughing?   Sneezing?   Lifting?   Changing position?

Do you have difficulty stopping the urine stream?

Do you experience incontinence at any of the following times:
When you are on the way to the restroom?
When you see or when you are near a restroom?
When you see or hear running water?
When you arrive home?
When you are nervous?

How often do you urinate during your waking hours?
How often do you awaken to urinate?

31

Incontinence & Pelvic Pain History
Page 2

Do you experience any of the following:
A weak urine flow?
Dribbling after voiding?
Urgency soon after you void?

With urination, do you have difficulty starting the stream?

Do you have difficulty voiding completely?

Do you experience pain with urination?

Do you have blood in your urine?

Do you have blood in your stools?

Do you sense urine in your bladder?
If yes, how long can you wait once you sense a full bladder?

Do you experience incontinence without being aware?

Do you sense urgency without emptying a full bladder?

Do you leak urine?   If yes, how much urine is lost?
Drops?   A full pad?   A cupful or more?

Do you wear protective undergarments?

How often do you move your bowels?

Do you experience diarrhea?   Or constipation?

Do you use a product or products to help move your bowels?
If yes, please name product(s):

Have you attempted Kegeling?

Figure 4: A general questionnaire presented upon intake.

Patient Questionnaire

Page 1

Name:
Age:
Date:

What is/are the condition(s) you would like addressed with physical therapy?

Please circle any of these medical conditions you currently have or previously have experienced:

High / Low blood pressure	High cholesterol	Heart disease
Peripheral artery disease	Muscle conditions	Asthma
Osteoporosis / Osteopenia	Pain in joints	Diabetes
Rheumatoid arthritis	Osteoarthritis	Stress
Pacemaker	Emphysema	

Other (please specify):

Previous surgeries:

Please list medications you are currently taking:

Please circle your current pain level:
0 (no pain) 1 2 3 4 5 6 7 8 9 10 (the worst pain)
Please state the pain level on your best day: and on your worst day:

What is your current level of function as compared to prior to the injury/condition?   %

Please circle the activities with which you are having difficulty?

House work	Childcare	Changing position
Yard work	Shopping	Negotiating stairs
Carrying	Walking	Keyboarding
Driving	Sitting	Sleeping
Exercising	Squatting	Lifting
Working (please specify)		
Other (please specify)		

Patient Questionnaire
Page 2

What are your goals for physical therapy?

Have you previously been treated in physical therapy for this condition?

Please list any other health professionals tending to your needs:

May we contact the above professionals if/when needed?

Please circle any diagnostic tests you have had for this condition?
MRI   EMG   X-ray   CT scan   Ultrasound
Other (please specify):

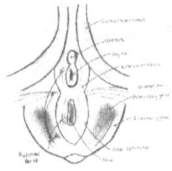

The Almighty Kegel: Contraction of the Pelvic Floor

The lack of pelvic floor muscle control is often a common denominator among several types of pelvic dysfunction. Learning to contract and relax the pelvic floor muscles can help resolve many conditions. In later sections, including *'Building the Kegel Strength from Zero to Hero'*, *'Stress Urinary Incontinence Rehabilitation Is Not "Just Kegeling"'*, and *'Patients with Stress Urinary Incontinence Trudged into My Care, but with Rehabilitation, They Danced Out'*, I will discuss the functional gains with specific scenarios I have treated. For now, I will provide an overview of this holy muscle contraction known as the 'Kegel'.

Contraction of healthy pelvic floor muscles results in stopping the urine stream. The contraction also engages in defecation prevention as well as intercourse. The pelvic floor muscles act to close the orifices of the perineum, or undersurface of the pelvic cavity.

When voluntarily and consciously contracting the pelvic floor, or Kegeling, we can often feel the contraction of the posterior (rear) muscles first, and the anterior (front) muscles second. The muscles seem to relax in the reverse order. The anterior muscles normally release first, the posterior muscles second. I speculate that the order of contracting and relaxing is a reason I have seen numerous cases of urinary incontinence instead of fecal incontinence. It appears to take more effort to contract the anterior muscles than to contract the posterior. It also seems more difficult to hold onto the contraction of the anterior muscles. Hence, between urinary and fecal control, urinary control appears to be the more difficult task, and the lack thereof has been the issue I have treated more frequently.

In the grand scheme of urinary control, the pelvic floor musculature ordinarily boasts 3 functional elements:

1. An automatic contraction responds to sensing urine in the bladder.
2. A voluntary contraction combats a strong, building urge to urinate, and prevents or halts an undesired urine stream.
3. A release of the muscle contraction allows for voiding when appropriate.[2]

We, as children, normally develop an automatic response to urinary urgency, which draws on the pelvic floor muscles to counter urine flow. The pelvic floor muscles can also be automatically called upon to stabilize the lumbar and pelvic regions to resist perturbation.[2] As we develop, we usually acquire pelvic floor muscle strength and agility from these automatic responses instead of from conscious contractions of these muscles. This differs from how we usually build muscles in other parts of the body. As children, we normally *learn* how to lift with our biceps, write and grasp with our hand muscles, and climb over a crib or fence using muscles in the legs and arms, and in the torso. These conscious actions can *actively train* the arm, leg, and torso muscles to perform specific functions and simultaneously build the muscles' strength and agility. Throughout our lives we can continue to consciously use these muscles and build their strength and agility with daily chores and exercise. We are normally well aware of these muscles especially when we lift, squat and jump. In contrast, we usually do not consciously train the pelvic floor to contract. As children, we are normally coaxed to find a restroom instead of soiling our undies! And, in due time, we seem to ignite the automatic response to control our urine flow successfully on a regular basis. Problems can arise, however, if the automatic responses are not enough to keep the pelvic floor muscles strong, or the muscles are over-strained or traumatized…then, a conscious effort to exercise the pelvic floor muscles may need to kick in!

"This is like learning how to walk!"

Our first successes at controlling urine flow can be compared to taking our first steps. Contracting the pelvic floor and walking are both automatic acts. Walking can even be thought of as a reflex: As the leading limb propagates forward, a stretch is applied to the hip flexor muscles of the trailing limb, and the hip flexors respond by contracting. The hip flexors' reflexive contraction lifts the trailing leg and moves it forward. Forward momentum is generated as we walk, and with successive steps we can repeatedly and reflexively "catch" ourselves from falling flat on our faces! We can tell ourselves to start moving, but, in healthy scenarios, we *do not have to think* about the actual walking motion. We can, however, actively control how fast our legs move. For example, normally if we are in a hurry, we can deliberately move our legs quickly. Similarly, in healthy scenarios, when the urine level rises above the half way mark in the bladder, we normally *do not have to think* about contracting of our pelvic floor muscles to keep our urine from flowing. In normal situations, we can automatically contract our pelvic floor muscles to "catch" our urine and prevent leaking. And, like forcing our legs to walk quickly when in a hurry, we can voluntarily force the contraction of the pelvic floor muscles when needed... But, we still may not know *exactly* where we are contracting, or how the pelvic floor muscles actually work! Despite not knowing exactly how or where we are contracting, we can still ordinarily tell ourselves to hold the pelvic floor muscles with everything they've got, as when the bladder feels like it is about to burst!! Therefore, in less extreme scenarios, the pelvic floor contraction is normally automatic, but when the bladder's detrusor is putting up a grand fight, a stronger, more cognizant contraction of the pelvic floor *can* be pulled into battle.

If we never actively or consciously set out to strengthen the pelvic floor muscles the first time around, *"retraining"* of the pelvic floor contraction is practically a misnomer. I prefer to tell patients that we are *training* the muscles to *re-engage* in countering urine flow and stabilizing the lumbar and pelvic regions, and *training* to release the contraction of muscles that may have become excessively tense and painful. *Training* the pelvic floor to contract is similar to teaching a patient to walk, since both acts were initially automatic responses. In fact, I often hear from patients, "This is like learning how to walk!" Grasping the concept of contracting a muscle we *never had to think about* can be very challenging! Initially such training is highly cerebral, and a concentrated effort is needed to contract the pelvic floor. With time, the response to the call for continence takes less and less of a conscious effort, and becomes more cerebellar if you will. With therapy, as I will explain in later sections, including *'Acquiring a Resting Tone in the Pelvic Floor Muscles'*, an extremely strong hold of the pelvic floor can ultimately be achieved for those emergency situations, a moderately strong baseline hold can be achieved for normal urges, and both can become automatic once again.

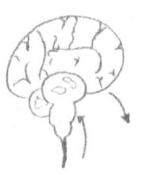

The Kegel's Resulting Neural Feedback

It is important to note that there are two muscles involved with incontinence that we cannot control *directly*: The detrusor muscle lining the bladder and the internal sphincter muscle where the proximal urethra meets the bladder. In normal situations, as the bladder fills with urine, the detrusor muscle is stretched. A stretch reflex occurs and the detrusor muscle contracts thereby pushing urine against the internal sphincter. The sphincter opens, urine proceeds through the urethra and voiding occurs.[6]

Though we cannot directly contract and relax the bladder's detrusor and the internal sphincter, we can control these smooth muscles *indirectly* via a feedback loop. Normally, contraction of the pelvic floor muscles sends a message to the brain's micturition center to halt voiding. From the brain, a message is sent to the stop the detrusor's contraction and to close the internal sphincter at the bladder's urethral opening. The relaxation of the pelvic floor muscles has the opposite effect. Without contraction of the pelvic floor, there is no a message to stop the contraction of the bladder. The bladder's detrusor muscle contracts when the bladder is moderately full and the internal sphincter opens. Therefore, although we are not directly contracting and relaxing the bladder's detrusor muscle or the internal sphincter around the urethra, we can control these muscles indirectly with a strong contraction or with relaxation of the pelvic floor. Under ordinary circumstances, a message to stop voiding is sent with a strong pelvic floor contraction, and the lack thereof results in reflexive voiding.[8,9] (See Figure 5a.)

Figure 5a. Illustration of the pelvic floor's feedback loop to the brain's micturition center and bladder.

The contraction of the pelvic floor muscles (bottom right) sends the message to the micturition center of the brain (upper left), which then signals the bladder (mid right) to stop contracting.

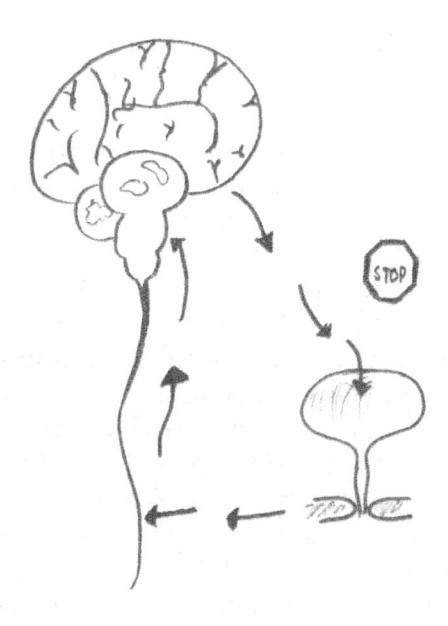

When the muscles of the pelvic floor are weak or are fatigued, their contractions may not provide adequate feedback to stop urine from flowing uncontrollably. On the other hand, an inability to relax the pelvic floor muscles can result in excessive signaling to hold the urine and a patient may have difficulty voiding. Both scenarios are quite common. These scenarios can also be combined. When a patient is unable to fully relax the pelvic floor muscles, the muscles may become fatigued. The muscles may hold strongly enough to make it difficult to fully void, but when a strong burst of a contraction is needed, as when countering the force of a sneeze or cough, they may be too tired to deliver. When the fatigued muscles fail to counter the extra force, urine escapes the bladder and incontinence befalls.

Better Start Kegeling...and Don't Forget to Release!

Training the pelvic floor helps to ensure healthy contraction *and* relaxation. The contraction can counter the urine flow by closing the external sphincter. Furthermore, the contraction can indirectly inhibit the detrusor's push on the internal sphincter by quieting the detrusor's contraction via the feedback loop. A moderate baseline tone can keep the pelvic floor on its toes, ready to hold against a push from the detrusor, and ready to feed into the message loop to dissuade a premature detrusor contraction and its emerging urinary urgency. When urination is not appropriate, proper conditioning can hold the urine in check and quell the bladder's force until voiding is indeed desired. When urination is appropriate and desired, adequate control can allow the pelvic floor muscles to fully release in order to urinate completely.

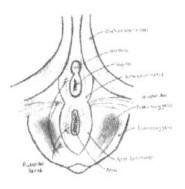

The Gateway to Pelvic Floor Control is the Isolation of Its Contraction

Oftentimes when patients attempt to Kegel to counter urine flow, they engage the abdominal muscles in conjunction with the pelvic floor muscles. This co-contraction is counterproductive. Adding the abdominals is like adding a cough or a sneeze. Like coughing and sneezing, contracting the abdominal muscles applies intra-abdominal pressure onto the bladder, which can cause the bladder to compress and the urine to leak. A compressed bladder can push urine forcefully into the urethra and make it difficult for the pelvic floor muscles to hold the external sphincter closed.

Imagining an attempt to keep a water hose from leaking by covering the nozzle with a thumb can put this co-contraction scenario in perspective. Preventing water from gushing out of an open-ended hose with a thumb requires the thumb's flexor muscles to hold it firmly in place over the nozzle. Stomping on the water-filled hose would create extra pressure in the hose and push the water more forcefully toward the thumb-covered nozzle. With excessive water pressure, water may seep or the thumb hold may fail completely. Co-contracting the abdominal muscles when attempting to Kegel is like stomping on the hose. The intra-abdominal pressure inherent in an abdominal muscle contraction can forcefully push the urine through the urethra, like the water being pushed through the hose. Urine rushing through the urethra can then overwhelm the pelvic floor muscles, like the water pushed by the stomping can overwhelm the thumb muscles. Overwhelming the pelvic floor by adding an abdominal contraction may therefore increase the chance of leaking urine and enhance the magnitude of an incontinent episode, rather than prevent one.

In addition to forcefully pushing urine through the internal sphincter, compressing the bladder can mimic the bladder's fullness and create an urgency to void. The sidewalls of the bladder's detrusor muscle can become stretched when the intra-abdominal pressure is applied downward from above. In response to this stretch, the bladder's detrusor muscle may reflexively contract and push urine through the internal sphincter. The pelvic floor muscles are therefore doubly taxed when a Kegel is accompanied by an abdominal contraction. They must hold against urine being pushed out of the bladder by the intra-abdominal pressure and against a detrusor muscle contracting in response to being stretched. These forces alone are difficult to counter, and together they can make holding a Kegel difficult or impossible. (See Figure 5b.)

Figure 5b. Comparison of the bladder without (top) and with (bottom) extra intra-abdominal pressure.

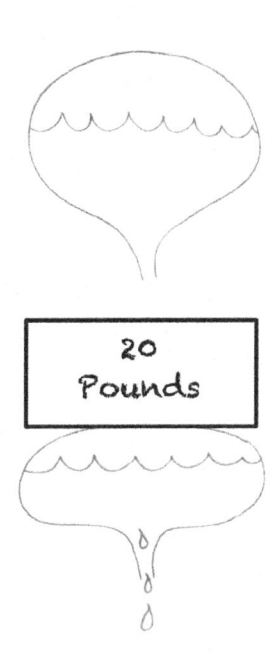

Some patients can isolate the pelvic floor from the abdominals, but only for a second or two, or only with a weak contraction. Once these patients attempt to contract for a longer period or with more force, the abdominals often engage. This level of endurance and amount of contractile strength of the pelvic floor are inadequate for countering incontinence on a regular basis.

Often in attempting to Kegel, some patients will also engage the adductor muscles of the inner thigh, which act to bring the legs together, and the gluteal muscles of the buttocks, which extend and rotate the hips. Some patients contract the adductors and gluteals in attempts to physically close the external urethral opening. Contraction thereof does not add intra-abdominal pressure, and can somewhat close the port. However, contracting the gluteals and especially the adductors is of no use when stepping to the side or getting out of a vehicle, whereby the legs are somewhat apart. It is therefore important to not rely on the gluteals and adductors, and instead strengthen the pelvic floor muscles with isolated Kegels for continence.

When performing in the clinic or practicing independently, I have the patient contract the pelvic floor muscles only as intensely and for as long as she can in isolation of the abdominals, gluteals, and adductors. Even if the intensity is minimal and even if the contraction time is barely a second, isolation is key. Only with isolation achieved are the intensity and length of hold effective shields against incontinence.

When training a patient to isolate the pelvic floor, I have her place a hand on the muscles that are interfering with isolation, i.e., abdominals, adductors, and gluteals. This way, she can feel when these accessory muscles are contracting and disengage them. An alternative means to promote an isolated contraction of the pelvic floor is practicing the contraction while lying prone. If the abdominals contract, the patient can feel her abdomen lift up off the table. Furthermore, in sitting, the patient can feel the altered seat pressure if she contracts the gluteals. Isolation of the pelvic floor is a difficult task for many patients. The pelvic floor contraction may have been performed in conjunction with the contraction of these outer muscles for quite some time, and often without the knowledge of such. With concentration and cues, the patient can achieve isolation. With proper training and practice over time, the co-contraction habit can break.

Practicing the isolated Kegel independently with a home exercise regime can expedite success. Finding the time to implement the true Kegel can be a challenge, but in due time, the exercises can and should be performed in conjunction with all activity! When using hands to determine whether the abdominals, adductors and/or gluteals are co-contracting, some patients prefer the privacy of their own homes. An excellent time to practice the isolated Kegel with hands in position to detect co-contractions, is right before going to sleep. Lying down to sleep is comfortable and the muscles of co-contraction infamy are easy to access. According to Hope, one of my patients treated for stress urinary incontinence, concentrating on her Kegels while lying down to rest was also an excellent way to unwind from a stressful day. Concentrating on the isolated Kegel cleared her mind of other distractions that had kept her from falling asleep for quite some time. By Kegeling, Hope was able to strengthen the pelvic floor muscles and drain her mind of stress…A Kegel meditation, if you will. Furthermore, Hope would often awaken about an hour before she actually had to rise. She found that the Kegels were easy to slide into her drowsy state and that they helped her to fall back to sleep! Thus, instead of counting sheep, she would count Kegels! A win win! Better sleep, and better pelvic floor control! (See Figure 6 for a bit of a giggle.)

Figure 6. Counting Kegels.

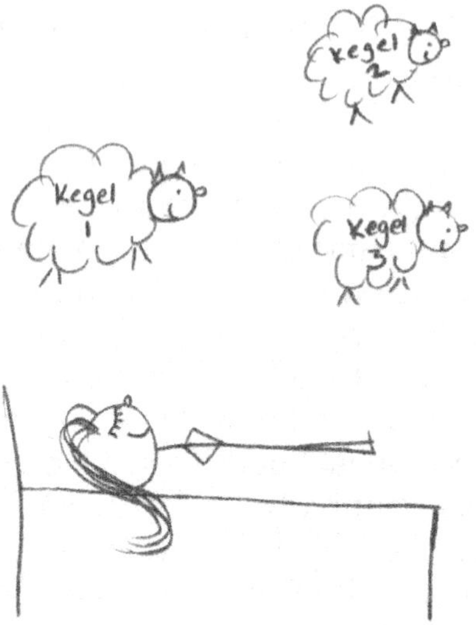

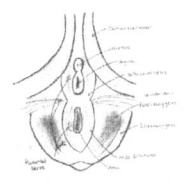

Helping Patients Find the Pelvic Floor Muscles

One difficulty I have come to find when training patients to restore the pelvic floor's strength is that patients cannot *see* the pelvic floor muscles contract. Patients are often unaware of the contraction when it is occurring naturally, as they do not *see* the muscles working. Patients sometimes are unaware that those muscles even exist! Training a patient to utilize muscles in the extremities and in the torso can often benefit from visual feedback rendered by the use of a mirror. Once the patient can *see* how she is to correctly perform an activity, she can attempt to perform the activity without visual cues and focus on *feeling the motion*. With progression, the patient can perform the activity without the need for visual feedback, and integrate the activity into her daily functions. Because visualizing the contraction of the pelvic floor is not practical, tactile cues and verbal cues are often used instead. The tactile and verbal cues may be less effective than visual feedback in general, but they can succeed in helping the patient grasp the concept of an isolated Kegel

Stopping the Urine Stream Once per Week

To introduce a Kegel, I often have a patient simulate an attempt to stop the urine flow. That is, in fact, what we are attempting to achieve in the realms of stress urinary incontinence and urinary urgency and frequency. I will often tell the patient to *test* the pelvic floor muscles once per week by commencing the urine stream, then stopping the flow midstream. With a successful Kegel, the patient can normally feel her pelvic floor muscles contract when the flow of urine slows or stops. This exercise can make use of the urine stream as a tactile cue and an audio cue, allowing the patient to feel and hear when she finds the muscles that control urinary flow.

Please note: I have always emphasized stopping the urine stream to test the pelvic floor's contraction *only once per week* because I do not want to confuse the micturition system and create or enhance a problem with fully voiding. I have not found the stopping and starting of urine flow as a contributor to difficulty voiding in the literature, but I certainly do *not* want to create grounds for it being there!

"Good thing I finally found you!"

After 13 years of telling countless patients to only test once per week, I finally came across a patient named Maura who shed light on my recommendation. Maura had difficulty keeping continent *and* fully emptying. When I recommended only stopping the stream once per week, she looked at me dumbfounded. "But I have been trying to stop the stream every day for years!" said Maura. "Even just after I use the restroom, I leak when I sneeze! Good thing I finally found you!" …I rest my case.

The Tampon Trick

A tampon partially inserted into the vagina can act as a tactile cue to help a patient sense where she is to contract in order to correctly perform a Kegel. The muscles that contract around the tampon and close the vagina belong to the pelvic floor. Contracting to close the vagina and hold the tampon can also close the external urethral sphincter and stop the urine flow. Therefore, despite the tampon contacting the vagina instead of the urethra, the tampon can act as a tactile cue telling the patient which muscles to contract when trying to keep from voiding. Once the contraction is achieved, gently tugging on the tampon while contracting the pelvic floor muscles can add resistance to the exercise...a *tug-of-war*, if you will.

The Pillow Trick

Sitting on a soft pillow or contoured cushion can also help patients "find" the pelvic floor muscles. This *pillow trick* can provide a tactile cue, whereby the soft pillow or contoured cushion pushes upward against the perineum, or undersurface of the pelvic floor. With the contraction of the pelvic floor muscles, a lifting sensation is often noted. The pillow's upward pressure on the perineum often lessens when the pelvic floor muscles contract. This is different from the sensation of lifting the entire buttocks off the chair as when contracting the gluteal muscles. With an isolated Kegel, only the pressure on the perineum changes. This change in pressure is a cue that the pelvic floor muscles have been found!

The *pillow trick* is the most versatile of the tools used to cue the pelvic floor's whereabouts. It is more readily available than the *tampon trick,* as it can be utilized *anywhere* a patient can sit. It can also be used *anytime* a patient can sit. The pillow trick can therefore render feedback as to when the pelvic floor muscles have been engaged on a more regular basis than stopping the urine stream, which should only be used once per week. Anywhere and anytime a pillow is available, the *pillow trick* can help patients find the pelvic floor muscles and integrate the Kegel into their day.

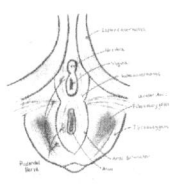

Building the Kegel Strength from Zero to Hero

At the beginning of therapy, I help the patient determine the length of time and the intensity at which to practice Kegeling. We determine the time she needs to find the pelvic floor muscles and how long she is able to hold in isolation. Finding the contraction may take a few seconds, but then attempting to hold for too long can result in the incorporation of the abdominals, adductors, and/or gluteals. Although the patient may be able perform a light contraction in isolation, she may take a turn for the worse when attempting to hold more firmly. Therefore, after finding the pelvic floor muscles, Kegels are to be performed only as long and as firmly as the patient can hold the contraction in isolation…Even if those first Kegels only last for a split second and exert only a flicker of strength. With practice, the time to find the muscles can drop, and the longevity of a strong, isolated contraction can improve.

In most of my cases of pelvic floor weakness, the patients have found it easiest to contract the pelvic floor in supine, or lying down on her back. In supine, the contents of the pelvic cavity are not fully weighing on the pelvic floor and fully pressuring the orifices to open. In sitting and even more so in standing, the contents' force on the pelvic floor can stretch apart the orifices like the mesh of a hammock that spreads when a person sits or lies on its threads. The lighter force in supine can make it easier for the pelvic floor muscles to close the orifices. Furthermore, in supine, the pelvic floor muscles do not have to work against gravity. (Standing on one's hands to Kegel would probably be the easiest of contraction attempts, but that task alone may pose a problem for some. Hanging upside down on a jungle gym or an inversion table may be better options to fully eliminate gravity.) Attempting to close the orifices with versus without the weight of the pelvic contents pressing downward to expand them can be compared to trying to bend an arm with versus without a weight in hand. Without weight, the biceps muscle contraction can normally move the arm into a bent position. However, when trying to lift a heavy object, the biceps can contract, but they may not be able to bend the arm due to the weight in hand being too heavy to lift. With the weight of the pelvic contents pressing downward to expand the orifices, the pelvic floor muscles can contract, but they may be unsuccessful in closing the orifices due to the "heaviness" of the load lying upon them. By providing a lighter force on the orifices and giving the pelvic floor muscles a good chance at contracting to close the external urethral sphincter, the supine position, versus sitting or standing, has allowed many patients to most easily perform their Kegels.

For many of my patients who have experienced difficulty "finding" the pelvic floor muscles, stopping the urine stream and utilizing the *tampon trick* and the *pillow trick* provided necessary guidance as to where they were to contract when performing a Kegel. The stream stopping and *tampon trick* can provide excellent cues, but these methods are not as easy to implement into a hectic day as the *pillow trick*. The tactile cue provided by the *pillow trick* is often just what some patients need in order to help them most easily perform a Kegel, making sitting on a pillow or contoured cushion their position of choice.

Aside from providing a sensation of lifting away from the chair, I speculate that sitting on a soft pillow or contoured cushion may actually help counter the force of the pelvic organs pressing on the pelvic floor…and, this may be why some patients find it easier to Kegel while sitting versus lying supine or standing. The weight of the pelvic contents can repeatedly bear down on the pelvic floor, over-stretching its muscle fibers. Excessive lengthening of the pelvic floor muscles can make them more difficult to contract. As I will elaborate on in a later section entitled '*Muscle Fiber Configurations Can Dictate Ease of Contraction, And the Lack Thereof*', excessive muscle fiber lengthening can create a weakened state whereby the muscle fibers cannot grasp optimally onto one another. Even in supine, with less weight on the pelvic floor, the muscle fibers may still be habitually overly lengthened due to childbirth or trauma. The counterpressure of the pillow or contoured cushion may reposition the muscle fibers in a configuration that provides them more strength. A visual that comes to mind is the Slinky, a toy popular with the children of the '70s and '80s. A Slinky being held at one end and left to drop at the other springs and stretches its coils. Once the springing stops, the coils are left in an overly lengthened position. A platform under the dangling coils can bring them back to their original state. Like the platform supporting the Slinky's coils, the pillow or contoured cushion may reposition the pelvic floor muscle fibers in an appropriately overlapped configuration. The pillow or contoured cushion may provide counterpressure against the downward force of the pelvic organs and keep the pelvic floor muscle fibers from overly lengthening like the platform can keep the Slinky from overstretching. By countering downward pressure and possibly keeping the pelvic floor muscle fibers in a position of advantageous length, sitting on a soft pillow or contoured cushion can give some patients their best chance at successfully contracting the pelvic floor.

Still for others, though rare, standing has been the position most conducive to performing the Kegel. These patients have told me that they can best *feel* the pelvic floor muscles working while they are standing versus sitting or lying supine. Perhaps the full weight of the pelvic contents pressing downward on the pelvic floor actually works in some patients' *favor*. Sensing the pelvic contents pressing against the pelvic floor can help patients realize where they are to contract. The sensation of pulling the full weight of the pelvic contents upward may give patients feedback that they are indeed performing a Kegel. This sense of a strong upward pull may be the cue some patients need, making standing the best position for these patients to Kegel.

To initially improve upon the isolated contraction, I help a patient find the position that most easily allows her to Kegel successfully. Once the isolation is achieved and the patient is confident in a performing a solid contraction, I then introduce more challenging positions. I challenge the patient to Kegel with activities such as rocking back and forth on uneven surfaces, standing with the legs abducted or separated laterally, and standing with one foot in front of the other. To progress, I challenge the patient to Kegel with activities such as ascending a step, walking, lightly jumping, high jumping, running, and swinging a racket or golf club. The Kegels can become more and more automatic as a patient learns to Kegel while performing other activities. Asking a patient to Kegel while simulating her daily activities helps her to implement the newly strengthened, automatic Kegel into her daily life. In subsequent sections, including '*Patients with Stress Urinary Incontinence Trudged into My Care, but with Rehabilitation, They Danced Out*', I will reveal in greater detail the progressive engagement of the pelvic floor's isolated contraction with examples of cases that have come into my care.

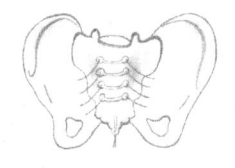

When Verbal and External Tactile Cues Are Not Enough, Give Biofeedback and Electrical Vaginal Stimulation a Try

Biofeedback utilizes an internally inserted, vaginal electrode to assist in determining whether or not a patient is contracting the pelvic floor muscles. A vaginal electrode looks like a short, stubby tampon. It is attached to an external biofeedback unit that generates visual and audible signals when the muscles surrounding the vaginal walls and urethra tighten around the electrode. (For men, there is a thinner, rectal electrode that signals contraction around the rectal walls.) The visual and audible cues allow a patient to see and hear how strong the contraction is, and how long she can hold the contraction. Without contracting, the resting tone of the pelvic floor muscles can be measured. All in all, biofeedback's visual and audio signals indicate the pelvic floor's magnitudes of contraction and relaxation.

When patients have difficulty finding the pelvic floor muscles, are unable to voluntarily contract against even a weak urine stream, or reach a plateau in strengthening, I suggest using electrical vaginal stimulation. I use the same type of electrode for the electrical vaginal stimulation as I do for the biofeedback. The electrode is inserted into the vagina by the patient and is connected to an electrical stimulation unit that is specifically designed for internal use, but remains outside of the body. The level of stimulation is controlled with a simple touch of a button. With the electrode inserted, I turn on the unit and slowly increase the intensity of the electrical pulses. The electrical stimulation is to be gentle and comfortable. Its intensity is to increase gradually as th e patient's vaginal walls become desensitized to the electrical pulses. A comfortable yet effective level of stimulation is established and the treatment proceeds.

With the electrode inserted and the electrical stimulation set to a comfortable level, I ask the patient to contract her pelvic floor muscles around the electrode. The patient holds the contraction or performs a series of short contractions while the stimulation is present and rests when the stimulation halts. The contraction and rest times cycle through for a preset period of time. A number of different settings are available for the treatment sessions. As I will elaborate on in subsequent sections, multiple duty cycles, or durations of stimulation and rest periods, and multiple stimulation frequencies allow for adequate muscle contraction and rest times with the frequencies best suited to treat the conditions at hand.

In their initial stages of rehabilitation, many of my patients found that Kegeling with the electrical stimulation became progressively *easier* over the course of 15 minutes, instead of more difficult with fatigue. This, I speculate, is because the patients initially needed successive stimulations to find the pelvic floor muscles and get a literal and figurative grasp of the contractions. Once these patients got a firm grip on the pelvic floor's contraction, they were able to contract with greater ease. With progressive treatment sessions of Kegeling with electrical stimulation, the patients were able to exert more force throughout the session. At this point they started noting fatigue over the course of 15 minutes. The electrical vaginal stimulation helped the patients secure a strong Kegel. The stronger the contractions, the more fatigued the muscles became with a 15-minute bout of stimulation-assisted contractions. With time and practice, however, the patients were able to sustain a series of strong Kegels over the course of 15 minutes, denoting Kegels of increased force *and* endurance.

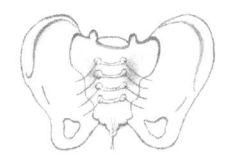

The Electrode and Electrical Stimulation

Tactile Stimulation

The electrode, with or without its emitted stimulation, can help a patient find the pelvic floor muscles with a tactile cue. Just inserting the electrode, even without electrical impulses, can direct a patient where to contract. At home, a patient can use the electrode to find the correct muscles merely by inserting it into the vagina and contracting around it, like performing the aforementioned *tampon trick*. Clinicians, let me explain with an analogy: For a patient relearning to engage the quadriceps when ascending a step, placement of the hands just above the knee can provide a tactile cue to contract the knee extensors which help propel the patient up the step. Similarly, the vaginal electrode can provide a tactile cue to enhance the contraction of the pelvic floor muscles and help resolve the weakness associated with a number of pelvic dysfunctions. In the clinic, the added electrical vaginal stimulation can enhance the tactile cue for an even greater sense of awareness. As previously mentioned, the initial development of the pelvic floor's contraction is automatic. Therefore, having a tactile cue to train *where* to *actively* contract has worked wonders for patients and has assisted clinicians in providing a means of successful rehabilitation.

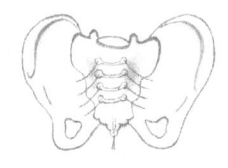

Electrical Stimulation in a Bit More Detail

Added Force of Contraction and Assisted Relaxation

When combined with the patient's active contraction, electrical vaginal stimulation can increase the muscle fibers' ability to forcefully contract the pelvic floor.[10] Clinicians, the effect of adding electrical vaginal stimulation for pelvic floor control is similar to adding electrical stimulation to the quadriceps to assist a patient who is recovering knee extension strength after having had a stroke or surgery. The vaginal electrode propagates a stimulus to help contract the pelvic floor, giving it an added dose of activation.[11] My patients have reported sensing a stronger, more deliberate Kegel when contracting with the stimulation than when contracting without it. For several of my patients, simultaneous electrical vaginal stimulation and active pelvic floor contraction provided the most effective means of strengthening the pelvic floor.

As mentioned in a previous section entitled *'Better Start Kegeling...and Don't Forget to Release!'* and in later sections including *'Incomplete Voiding'* and *'Pelvic Pain'*, gaining control of the pelvic floor not only means a stronger contraction, it also means learning to release the hold of the muscles especially when excessive muscle tension is the culprit of pelvic dysfunction. A high stimulation frequency can actually assist in relaxing the pelvic floor muscles.[12] Helping the muscles relax can provide necessary recovery time and ease painful tension. This painful tension is often the cause of pain with intercourse and with an inability to completely void. During a treatment session with high frequency stimulation, the patients focus on relaxing instead of contracting. For many of my patients, the high frequency electrical vaginal stimulation has helped release their overly exerted muscles, and the ensuing muscle recovery has assisted in restoring their pelvic floor's muscle integrity.

Unfortunately, I have not found a means of testing the force of contraction whilst administering the stimulation simultaneously, as there can only be one device attached to the electrode at any given time. How do I know it works? Listening to the patients' subsequent subjective reports after having used the stimulation versus having not, and using biofeedback intermittently to test the contraction and resting tone before and after stimulation.

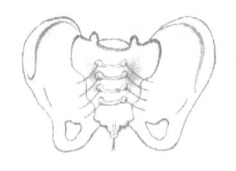

Electrical Stimulation Can Awaken the Pelvic Floor

After therapy sessions with electrical vaginal stimulation, patients have reported a heightened awareness of the muscles surrounding the vagina and urethra. Such a sensation can assist patients in *finding* these muscles independently when performing their home exercises, and more importantly when putting the Kegel to functional use to control urination! I have found that a lot of patients begin to independently *feel* where they are to contract after approximately three treatments with electrical stimulation. I call this an *awakening* of the pelvic floor. For cases of painful intercourse, this awakening has provided heightened sensitivity of the vaginal walls in a positive way. This sensitivity has correlated with improved production of natural vaginal secretions and tension release during intercourse, both of which have significantly improved patients' sexual experiences to a point where I have deemed the effects of their stimulation a *revival*. For many patients, this awakening or revival is an integral part of resolving pelvic dysfunction. I have been told by many of my patients that resolving such dysfunction had been monumental in overcoming the emotional distress of an integral part of their relationships that had gone amiss. With pelvic pain, intercourse can be a burden. Treatment not only has the potential to bury that burden, it can also revive a pleasurable experience!

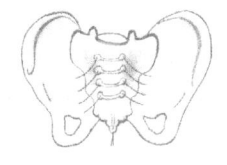

A Few Similarities and a Few Differences between Electrical Stimulation and Biofeedback

My approach to conducting biofeedback and internal electrical stimulation is hands-off. My patients insert and remove the vaginal electrode themselves. I find that this not only makes the patient more comfortable, it also moves the patient toward taking independent control of her pelvic floor's condition.

It is important to note that use of the electrode is contraindicated at times, such as with pregnancy, menses, infection, and with the use of pacemakers. For patients with pacemakers, there is a magnet that can be applied over the pacemaker to counter the adverse effects of the electrical stimulation. The use of the magnet with the electrical stimulator needs to be cleared by the patient's cardiologist. The patient and clinician must openly discuss the conditions that contraindicate the use of electrical stimulation, or even contraindicate the use of the electrode alone. When contraindicated, using the electrode with or without the stimulator could create a much more serious condition than the pelvic dysfunction it was meant to treat.

Of the two, I find electrical stimulation to be the more effective treatment. Biofeedback can tell the patients when, how long, and how strong they are contracting, and it can suggest a level of resting tone. However, my reasoning for electrical stimulation's prowess over biofeedback is three-fold. One, with electrical stimulation, patients can attain a heightened sense of where the pelvic floor muscles are. Two, with a boost of stimulation to the muscles, the patients can create a more powerful contraction and the Kegel muscles can get a more intense workout! Lastly, three, the pelvic floor's pent up tension can be relieved and its sensitivity revived. Both biofeedback and stimulation can be effective treatments, but in my opinion time is better spent with stimulation as it can yield a greater number of rehabilitative benefits all at once.

Muscle Fiber Configurations Can Dictate Ease of Contraction, And the Lack Thereof

The magnitude and ease of a pelvic floor muscle contraction is dependent on the length-tension relationship of its constituent muscle fibers. (See Figure 7a.) Muscle fibers form a line and partially overlap one another, grasping onto the fiber fore and aft with an interlocking mechanism. Over-lengthening a muscle affords only a small number of interlocking sites among its fibers. This minimal number of individual connecting sites works to its fullest capacity just to achieve a relatively weak contraction. This is why we would give our friend attempting to climb over a wall or reach a high tree branch "10 fingers" of support by interlocking at the base of our fingers instead of at our fingertips. If we grasp only with our fingertips, our finger hold can fail. Similarly, if muscle fibers are overly lengthened, the muscle's overall contractile force is at a disadvantage.[13]

Shortening the overall muscle length (contracting) can be advantageous to contractile strength, but only to a point.[13] Cramping can occur at extremely shortened configurations, which can lead to pain and muscle failure. Such pain can make it difficult to voluntarily contract the muscles. If we fully flexed or bent our fingers whilst providing "10 fingers", they could become uncomfortably tense. Our "10 fingers" would then likely give way and fail at providing a base of support. An overly shortened configuration among the pelvic floor muscle fibers can also create pain and cause the pelvic floor to fail to fulfill its responsibilities.

Another analogy that may help to understand the length-tension relationship involves a simple pull-up. To start a pull-up with elbows in a fully straightened position (from a "dead hang") can be very challenging. To pull with the elbows flexed or bent halfway may not be as difficult. That final pull up and over the bar when the elbows are nearly fully flexed can pose quite a challenge. The "dead hang" can overly lengthen the biceps. The midrange positions are mechanically advantageous, but only until that last bit of flexion or bending is needed to complete the pull-up. (See Figure 7b.)

The same can be said for attempting a Kegel as attempting a pull-up. With the pelvic floor muscles in a semi-contracted position, the Kegel is likely most effective. The pelvic floor muscles may assume an overly lengthened position when the legs are outstretched as when taking large steps, or abducted as when standing with the feet apart. In these positions, the contraction of the pelvic floor muscles can be quite challenging, or the attempt to contract may utterly fail. On the other end of the spectrum, contracting the pelvic floor musculature can also be a challenge when its muscle fibers are excessively shortened and cramped. Therefore, it appears as though when the muscle fibers are semi-overlapped, the muscles of the pelvic floor are easiest to contract. Outside of the mid-range lengths, the muscle fibers may struggle just to *hold on*, or angrily refuse to work due to cramping and painful tension.

Figure 7a. A graph of the length-tension curve.[13]

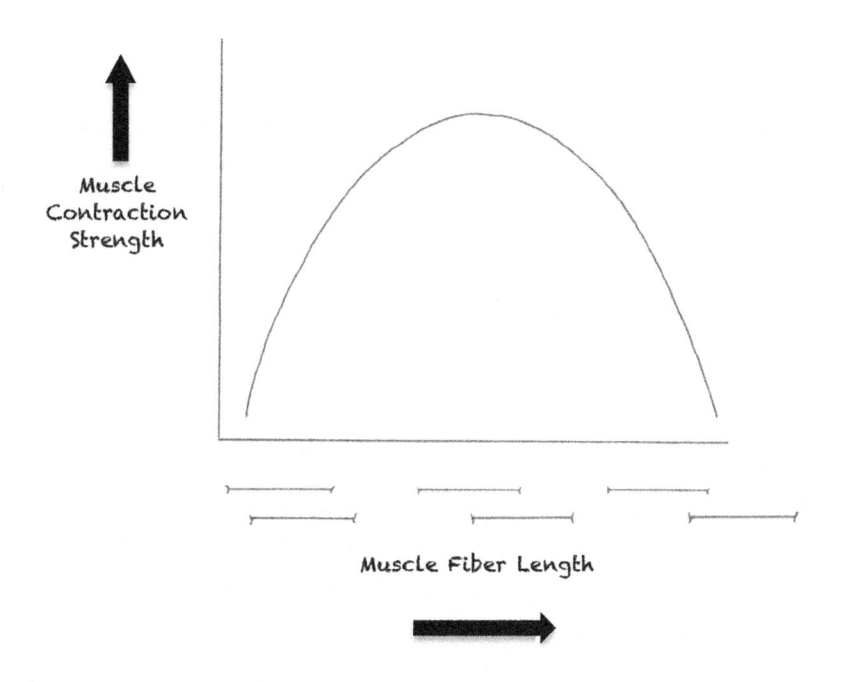

Muscle Contraction Strength ↑

Muscle Fiber Length →

Figure 7b. An analogy depicting exertion compared to muscle fiber length.

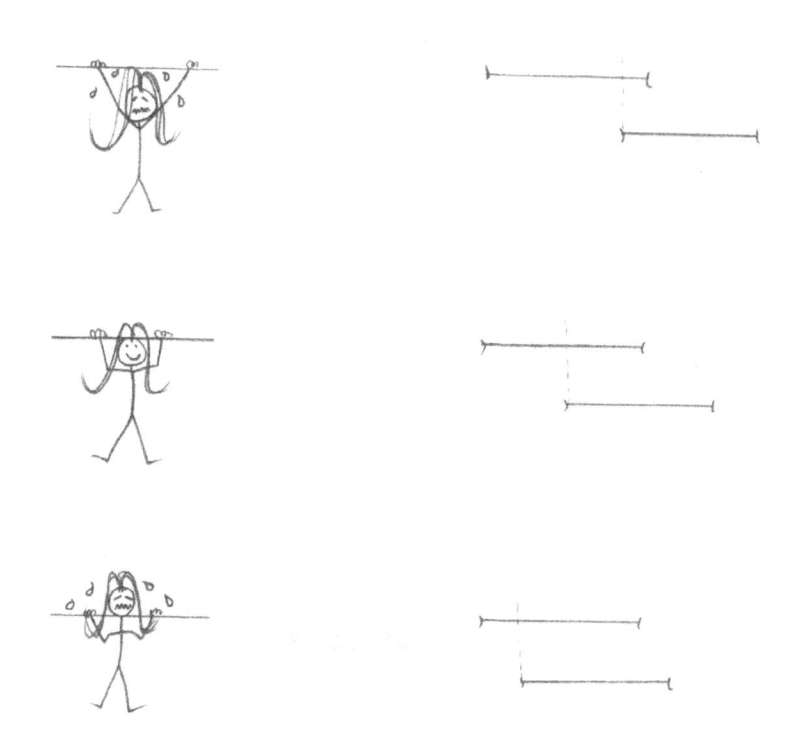

Muscle Fiber Length

Asymmetries Often Underlie a Mechanical Disadvantage of the Pelvic Floor

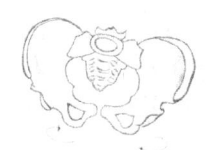

Altered length-tension relationships may correlate with pelvic and sacral asymmetries. These asymmetries occur when one side of the pelvis is higher or rotated more forward than the other, or when the sacrum is tilted. The pelvic and sacral presentations are referred to as elevations in the frontal plane (which divides the body's front side from the back), rotational asymmetries in the sagittal plane (which divides the body into left and right sides), and outflares and inflares in the transverse plane (which divides the upper body from the lower). Asymmetries can lead to *and* perpetuate inadequate pelvic floor muscle strength in a vicious cycle. With a strong Kegel being a key component of the core's contraction, weak pelvic floor muscles may hinder stabilization of the spine and pelvis. This instability can perpetuate asymmetries, which can create an environment of overly lengthened muscle fibers and intensify the difficulty of performing a Kegel.

The most common presentation of pelvic asymmetry I have seen in conjunction with incontinence is ilial elevation, whereby one side of the pelvis is raised in relation to the other. Why is this presentation so common? I speculate that the habitual standing posture with one hip protruding laterally (out to the side) and superiorly (upward), and walking with a hip sway can lead to and/or perpetuate the elevation. Holding children or objects on a hip in order to use the opposite hand to multitask, or even standing with one hip elevated due to fatigue or habit can promote tension in the low back muscles on the same side as the elevation or sway. These muscles can become shortened and eventually hold the pelvis in the elevated position. In addition, falling onto one side, ligamentous laxity with menses, and childbirth can all initiate the elevation. The habitual side-bent posture can perpetuate the elevation. The muscle fibers of the pelvic floor can consequently creep into overly lengthened positions and challenge the pelvic floor's muscle contraction. (See Figure 8.)

Figure 8. An illustration of ilial elevation and the correlating of pelvic floor muscle fiber length.

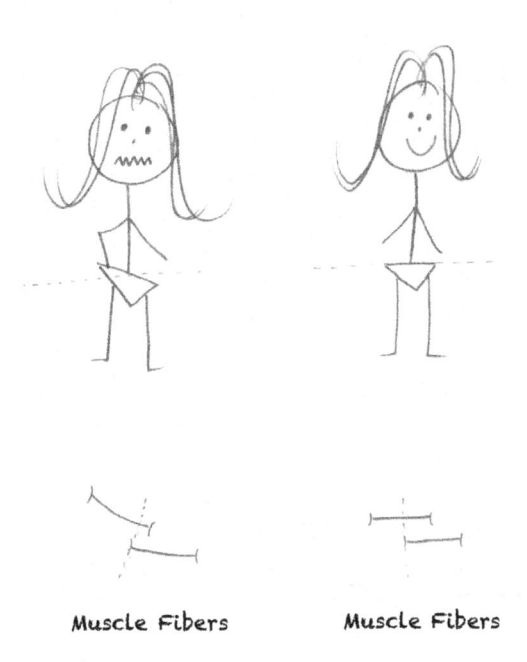

Muscle Fibers   Muscle Fibers

I have seen numerous cases of such ilial (side of pelvis) elevations with the likes of scoliosis, degenerative disc disease, and herniated and bulging discs. Scoliosis can create a curvature of the spine so great that in order to stand erect, one ilium or side of the pelvis elevates to counter the curvature. With lumbar disc degeneration, the withering away of the disc is very often asymmetrical whereby the one side of the disc degenerates to a greater degree than the other. Similarly, a herniated or bulging disc is like a water balloon being flattened on one side and enlarged on the other. The ensuing height differentials within the discs often create a shift in one side of the pelvis to compensate for the asymmetrical disc heights, similar to the scoliosis scenario. (See Figure 9.)

Sadly, these examples of length-tension alterations can lead to, and perpetuate, pelvic floor inadequacies by contributing to the disadvantageous over-lengthening of the pelvic floor muscle fibers. Hindering pelvic floor muscle control can render it less effective in countering the disorders of the pelvic region and stabilizing the spine and pelvis. Stabilizing the spine can minimize the progression of scoliosis and spinal degeneration, and can minimize further bulging and herniation of the spinal discs. Stabilizing the pelvis can minimize its asymmetries. Essentially, the pelvic floor strength helps to keep the integrity of the spinal segments and pelvis in check. But, malalignments caused by these very spinal conditions and habitual postures can make contracting the pelvic floor muscles difficult by disadvantageously lengthening its constituent muscle fibers. Therefore, a conscious effort to rehabilitate the spinal degradation and pelvic asymmetries is paramount to restoring pelvic floor integrity, and overall spinal and pelvic health.

Figure 9. An illustration of ilial asymmetries emerging from scoliosis, disc degeneration, and disc herniation or bulge.

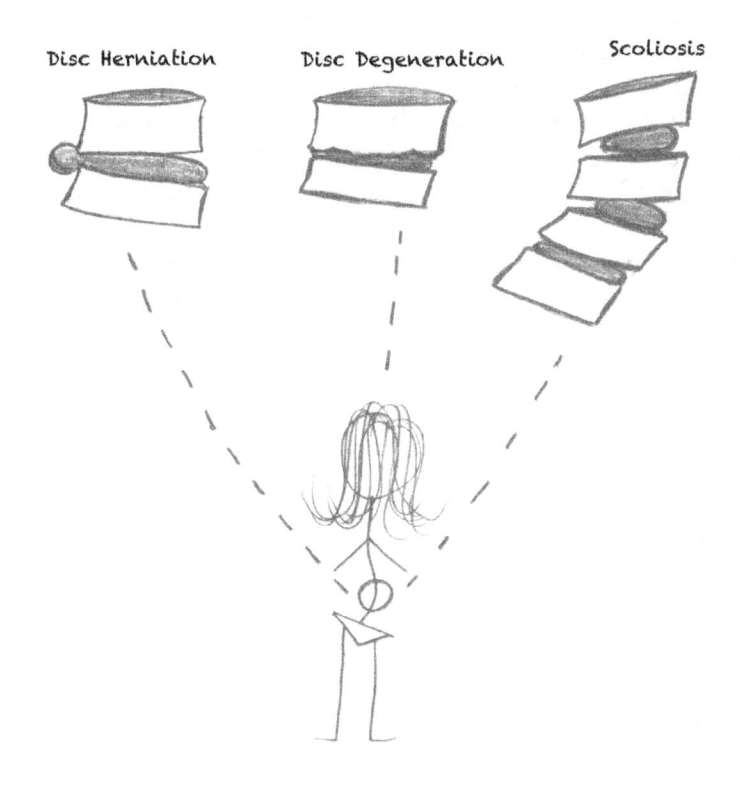

Disc Herniation   Disc Degeneration   Scoliosis

   Ilial (side of pelvis) asymmetry may stem from restricted muscles that attach to, or originate on, the pelvis. Muscle restrictions due to overuse and inadequate stretching often contribute to, or perpetuate, elevations, rotations and outward and inward pulls on the pelvis. All of these asymmetries can cause inadequately aligned pelvic floor muscle fibers. If the lumbar (low back) muscles, such as the quadratus lumborum, are restricted, the ilium it attaches to may be pulled upward or elevated. When the hamstring muscles are significantly more restricted or shortened on one side versus the other, they can create a posterior (backward) rotation of the respective side of the pelvis to which they are attached. If a hip flexor, such as the iliopsoas, is restricted on one side, it can pull its respective side of the pelvis anteriorly or forward. Inflares and outflares of the ilia can occur if hip rotators are restricted. The muscles that rotate the hip outward create a relative inflare of the ipsilateral, or same, side of the pelvis. Outflares occur in those with an internally rotated hip due to restricted, shortened hip internal rotators on the ipsilateral, or same, side. Please note, with all the flares and rotations, the side that is out of alignment is relative to the other, creating the opposite condition on the opposite side. All of the asymmetries may contribute to pelvic dysfunction and perpetuate their own contortions by weakening the pelvic floor's muscle fiber configuration. (See Figures 10a, 10b, and 11.)

Figure 10a. Anterior rotation of one ilium (side of pelvis).

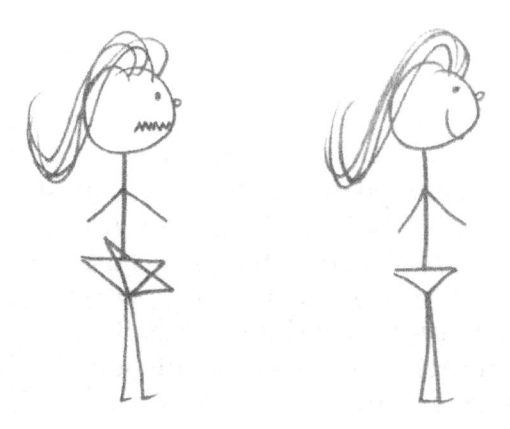

Figure 10b. A comparison of anteriorly rotated, posteriorly rotated, and neutral ilia (sides of pelvis).

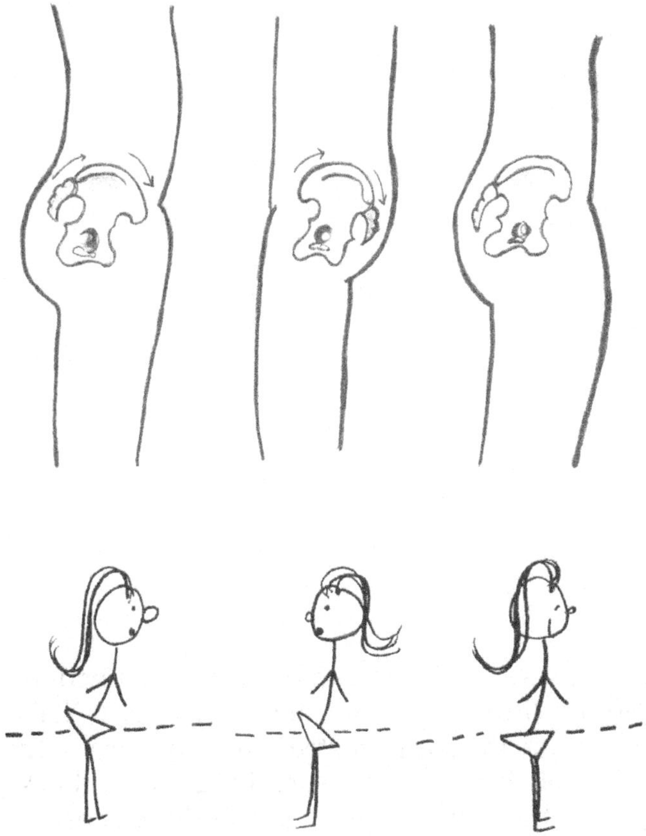

Figure 11. A depiction of an outflare of right-sided ilium (right side of pelvis), and an inflare of left-sided ilium (left side of pelvis).

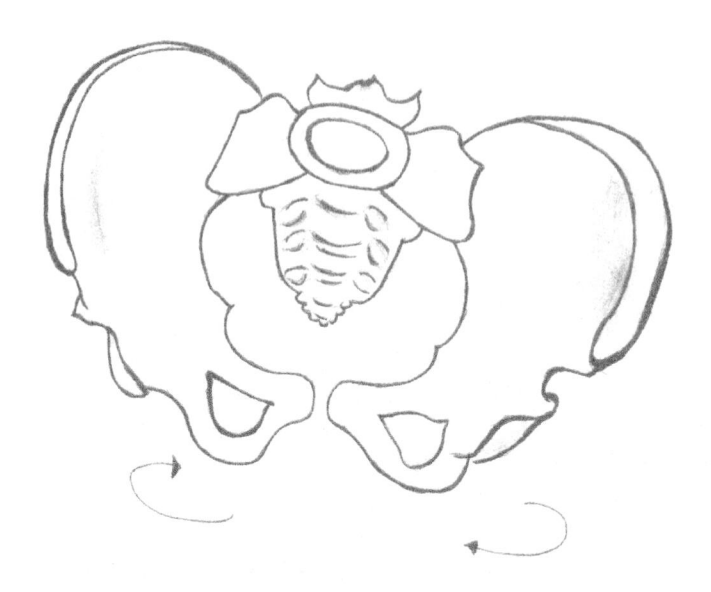

    Ligamentous laxity can occur in conjunction with multiple conditions and natural bodily cycles. This laxity can undermine the support structures that are needed to hold the lumbar, pelvic, and sacral regions in check. Falling onto the pelvic region may shift the constituent bones out of place, stressing the ligaments crossing the joints. Furthermore, the recurrent release of the relaxin hormone during the menstrual cycle and with use of oral contraceptives[14] can decrease the ligaments' holding power to support the lumbar, pelvic, and sacroiliac (where the sacrum meets the pelvis) joints. In order to prepare for pregnancy, the pelvis can expand in width with the help of the relaxin hormone. The influx of relaxin, like overstretching ligaments with a fall, can predispose the rearing of the ilial asymmetries. Asymmetries that may occur with ligamentous laxity can set a stage for disadvantageous pelvic floor muscle fiber configurations.

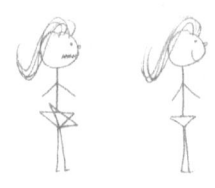

Treating Pelvic Asymmetries

In treating pelvic asymmetries and sacroiliac joint dysfunction, I have found it helpful to manually relieve tension in the muscles that are pulling the joints out of alignment, such as the quadratus lumborum in the low back, the hip flexors, and the hip rotators. It is also important to stretch the muscles surrounding the hips and pelvis to keep a neutral position of the muscle fibers. With less tension, osteopathic techniques can then gradually and isometrically pull the ilia (sides of pelvis) and sacrum into alignment. Stabilization is needed for the malalignment's resolution and minimal recurrence. A well-defined home exercise program should be developed to complement the clinician's techniques. The home program can give the patients the power to realign their own ilia (sides of pelvis) should the asymmetries recur, and the ability to progressively stabilize their alignment so they don't!

The most effective means of stabilizing I have encountered is activation of the true core comprised of the pelvic floor muscles and the deep abdominal muscle, known as the transverse abdominis. (The diaphragm is also a constituent of the true core, which is engaged with breathing.) Combining use of the pelvic floor with the abdominals gets tricky when pelvic asymmetries or sacroiliac joint dysfunctions are intertwined with stress urinary incontinence. Why? Because abdominal pressure created by transverse abdominis contraction can mimic a cough or a sneeze and can perpetuate incontinence. Furthermore, remember that the isolated contraction is key to ultimate control over the pelvic floor muscles. Adding an abdominal contraction can confuse the patient and worsen incontinence.

The very pelvic asymmetries that make it difficult to contract the pelvic floor, though, need stabilization. So what is a patient to do? I have found that patients are most successful when they learn to isolate the pelvic floor first, in order to control continence, and then train the full core to stabilize. The therapist can assist with realigning the pelvis during the treatments and provide self-help techniques in a home exercise program. The isolated pelvic floor contraction can at least partially stabilize the low back, pelvis, and sacrum as it brings stress urinary incontinence to an end. Once an isolated pelvic floor contraction is learned and successfully applied to countering incontinence, the transverse abdominis (deep abdominal) contraction can be introduced for full core control.

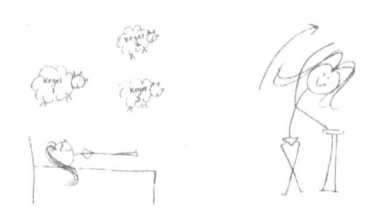

The Importance of a Home Exercise Program (...For Starters)

Before elaborating on the treatments for pelvic disorders, I would like to stress the importance of a home exercise program. Successfully rehabilitating all pelvic concerns, like other types of diagnoses, is heavily dependent on a patient's carryover of sound techniques and exercises into activities of daily living. I will address details of home programs in subsequent sections, including *'Tackling Stress Urinary Incontinence in a Bit More Detail'*, specifying self-help mechanisms pertaining to respective cases and conditions. Each case is unique, but one commonality applies to all: Not only can a home program reinforce strength, alignment, and neuromuscular integrity; it can also empower patients to take control of their conditions. A home program built to give patients the ability to sense a problem and the tools to fix it can instill confidence that pelvic dysfunctions can be controlled or resolved. The home exercise program is a means to help patients help themselves. So often patients do not want to even leave their homes due to the fear of urinating uncontrollably or sensing immense pain in public. Giving a sense of control can begin to chip away at this fear, restoring a life with less pain and greater pelvic function.

It is imperative that patients continue to perform the Kegel exercises and other prescribed self-help techniques even beyond their days of therapy. The pelvic floor muscles can respond like all muscles in that without exercise, their strength and agility can diminish.[15] I often tell patients that performing the home program is like brushing their teeth: Just as neglecting their teeth invites cavities, stopping the self-help can invite a relapse of pelvic dysfunction.

Incontinence

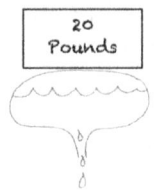

Stress Urinary Incontinence (SUI)

Stress urinary incontinence (SUI) is aptly named because when physical *stress* on the pelvic floor overwhelms pelvic floor muscles' contractile abilities, it can lead to involuntary urinary leakage. Sneezing, coughing, laughing, changing position, catching a ball, running, or otherwise jolting the torso can increase pressure intra-abdominally, which applies a force on the bladder. Such a force can simulate contraction of the detrusor muscle, whereby the urine presses forcefully against the internal sphincter and the external sphincter. With greater pressure applied to the pelvic floor muscles, their constituent fibers have to work harder to hold the external sphincter closed. Holding the external sphincter closed is just like trying to keep our fingers interlocked when our friend steps downward on our aforementioned step made of "10 fingers". Without a strong hold, the step fails. Without a strong pelvic floor, the external sphincter opens and voiding control is lost. (See Figure 12.)

Figure 12. Intra-abdominal pressure on the bladder and the ensuing void.

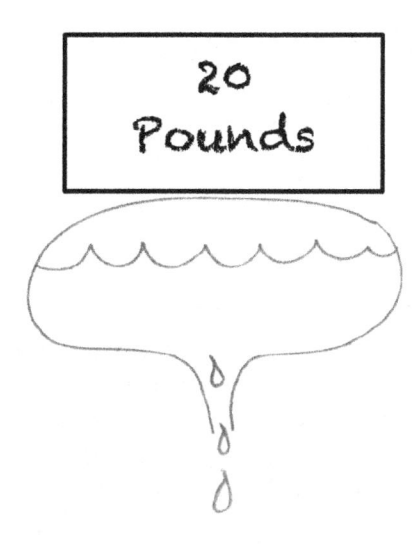

Treating stress urinary incontinence involves training the muscles surrounding the external sphincter to contract against urinary flow with the performance of a Kegel. (See Figure 13.) As I previously stated, to assist in learning a truly isolated Kegel, I may ask a patient to attempt to stop urine flow while urinating. I will re-emphasize here that I recommend patients perform this *only one time per week*. Again, I do not want to create a problem with fully voiding, a condition that will be discussed further in a later section entitled '*Incomplete Voiding*'.

Figure 13. A depiction of stress urinary incontinence and continence.

On the left, an inadequate pelvic floor muscle contraction leads to incontinence. On the right, a strong pelvic floor muscle contraction counters intra-abdominal pressure and prevents urination.

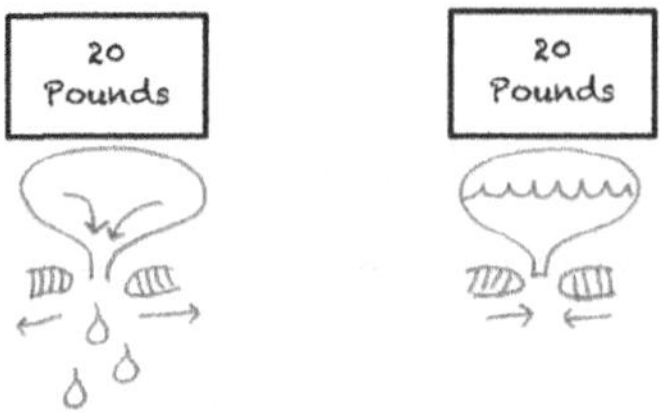

The aforementioned *tampon trick*, whereby a patient contracts the muscles that surround a partially inserted tampon, can cleverly cue the patient to correctly contract the pelvic floor. To progress beyond the weekly stopping of the urine stream and the initial *tampon trick*, I ask the patient to pull on the tampon string with her fingers when squeezing around the partially inserted tampon and, as previously described, play *tug-of-war* with the tampon. These *tampon tricks* can cue the patient where to contract and strengthen the muscles that can counter the unwanted urine flow.

Should active muscle contraction need assistance in combatting stress urinary incontinence, 50 Hz electrical vaginal stimulation can work wonders![11] As previously mentioned, the electrode can tactilely stimulate the pelvic floor muscles and the electrical stimulation can help activate the muscles to contract with greater conviction. With the electrical stimulation on, the patient contracts the pelvic floor muscles around the electrode, with all efforts made to contract in isolation of the gluteal, abdominal, and adductor muscles. I commonly set the stimulator to a duty cycle of 10 seconds on and 10 seconds off for a period of 15 minutes. If greater rest is needed between periods of contraction, I set the stimulator's rest period to 20 seconds. I keep the electrical stimulation on for 10 seconds even if the patient is not able to contract for the entire time. If the patient is only able to contract for 3 seconds, she can rest for a bit then re-engage the contraction for the remainder of the 10-second on time. With successive treatments, I find that the patient is not only able to contract for longer and longer periods, she is able to do so more strongly in isolation of the gluteal, adductor, and abdominal muscles. With the tactile cue and electrical activation, the patient can gain a better grasp of the pelvic floor's whereabouts and a stronger force of isolated contraction. Both of which pave the way to achieving continence.

When implementing electrically stimulated contractions, I recommend starting simply, then progressing to the challenge of multitasking. I recommend starting the treatments of electrical vaginal stimulation in supine. To progress, I suggest performing the electrically stimulated contractions in a multitude of positions such as standing, sitting, and standing with legs abducted or apart. To further challenge the patients, I suggest tossing a ball and walking with the electrically stimulated contraction surrounding the activity. Progressions such as these have granted successful carryover into contracting with activities in everyday life.

I have utilized biofeedback to evaluate the intensity of a patient's contractile strength, and to re-evaluate the contraction's force after a series of treatments and home exercises have been implemented. The force of contraction is useful to know. However, we must make the best use of time in the treatment session and, as I have previously mentioned, I recommend stimulation over biofeedback. The best "biofeedback", in my opinion, is the level of a patient's continence. That continence is faster achieved with a faster gain in strength using electrical stimulation as a catalyst.

It is imperative to note that, although adding electrical stimulation can enhance the pelvic floor's contraction, the actual Kegel itself is the shield against stress urinary incontinence. Kegel performance with the stimulation has been shown to outshine stimulation alone.[10] If there is no effect or a very slow effect of Kegeling alone, adding the stimulation while performing the Kegel can kick the muscles into gear. After the muscles are strong enough to start to counter intra-abdominal pressure and stop urine flow, the stimulation can add a focus and an extra burst of activation for overall strengthening. The holy Kegel is the foundation upon which functional gains are eventually made, and electrical stimulation can help build that foundation faster.

To complement treatments, I try to make it easy for patients to implement independent pelvic floor exercises into their day. Asking a patient to practice long holds and a series of shorts holds is a good starting point. A home program consisting of long, 10-second Kegels, 10 times per day, and 10 quick Kegels, 10 times per day helps to enhance pelvic floor strength. The number of sets appropriately matches the patient's level of strength and endurance. Once the patient can find the pelvic floor muscles without the use of a tampon or electrode for tactile stimulation, she can essentially perform her exercises anywhere…and no one will know that she is doing so. Performing a Kegel while sitting at a stop light, fueling a vehicle, standing in line at a store, getting into and out of bed, and walking to retrieve the mail are all means by which the patient can perform the exercises throughout her day without having to set aside a separate time for them.

Several articles of literature support the pelvic floor exercises as an effective treatment. One study involved several female soldiers who had experienced stress urinary incontinence in the field and noted success in achieving continence with Kegel exercises.[16,17] To fully rehabilitate, however, I find that recovery usually does not happen with just Kegeling alone. Without practicing the actual contraction in a functional setting, the strength gained while contracting with or without tactile stimulation or electrical stimulation goes to waste. As I will elaborate on in the next section, timing, endurance, and automaticity of the isolated contraction are all ingredients to successful continence in day-to-day life!

I have not asked patients to try vaginal weights. They are welcome to do so. However, if the patient cannot hold a particular weight, it will fall out and land on the floor or possibly land on a toe (ouch!). Cleaning the weights adds another step to the home exercise program. Furthermore, to use the weights, the patient needs a specific time and place to perform the exercises. I find the most effective means of helping to ensure a patient will perform an independent exercise program is making it as easy as possible to implement. The tampon tricks can be performed just after using the bathroom. The repeated contractions can be (and should be) performed anywhere! I respect the busy lifestyles my patients live. The performance of Kegels with any activity, regardless of where patients are and what they are doing, can make efficient use of time *and* integrate the Kegel into daily life.

With Kegeling, the pelvic floor muscles can become strong, but the road to continence does not end there. Once patients can isolate the muscles and strongly contract them, they must apply this strength in a functional manner, and gradually build a resting tone. Patients must then maintain a healthy resting tone and maintain the ability to react when continence calls. Allow me to elaborate…

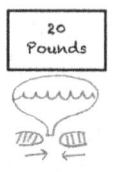

Timing is of the Essence

Stress Urinary Incontinence Rehabilitation Is Not 'Just Kegeling'

I emphasize to patients that full continence is not attained by 'just Kegeling' alone. Yes, achieving a true, isolated, strong Kegel is the groundwork, the foundation. It is indeed necessary to practice long strong holds, short strong holds, and long holds of moderate intensity with short bursts of force. However, if this strength is not implemented effectively, the acquired contraction will not resolve incontinence. The same is true of a person wanting to learn to swim. Solely strengthening the shoulder muscles in the gym is not enough. Without implementing that strength into a powerful and effective stroke, the person will likely sink. By adapting the strength into such a stroke, the person can learn to swim. Training to build power, endurance, reactive timing, and agility, all in a multitude of positions can yield a strong pelvic floor. The person who integrates this strength into daily activities can resume the timely automaticity of the pelvic floor's contraction and overcome incontinence.

There is a challenge to performing Kegels while performing activities of daily living. To assist in recovering the pelvic floor's automatic contraction, I ask patients to perform a wide range of tasks while Kegeling. Performing the contraction while distracted by another task such as catching a ball, walking, and biking, can help patients to associate the contraction with activities in their daily lives, and help make the contraction more automatic.

Timing the pelvic floor contraction *around* an activity is imperative to controlling urine's flow, and this timing is supported by literature.[18] Successful continence requires pelvic floor contraction before and during a sneeze, a cough, a bout of laughter, a change of position, and even a step. I advise patients to hold longer than the activity time to ensure success. If a second sneeze sneaks up, one must be ready to counter the second rush of intra-abdominal force! Therefore, Kegeling before, during, and for a short while after an activity can restore life without sneaky leaks!

I teach Kegel timing in a series of steps. First, before the start of an activity, I ask the patient to engage an isolated pelvic floor contraction. While continuing to hold the Kegel, the patient performs an activity such as standing from sitting. Only after the activity is fully complete is the patient to release the pelvic floor muscles. The patient can progress to holding the contraction through multiple, consecutive sit-to-stand-to-sit repeats. Even if the patient releases the contraction out of fatigue, I ask her to at least *think* about holding. This can reinforce the timing of the Kegel before, throughout, and for a short while after the activity, even if the muscles lack the endurance to uphold the contraction. Once endurance is achieved, the idea of contracting around the activity can then more quickly become second nature.

The timing process may begin at a slow pace. The patient may need time to concentrate on Kegeling first. While continuing to hold, she performs an activity that slowly adds intra-abdominal pressure. Activities that add a controlled force include slowly pulling a swim cord or therapy band and slowly pressing both hands onto a therapy ball. These exercises can then be performed multiple times, and with progressively longer holds, all the while emphasizing the timing of the Kegel.

Progress continues when the patient can quickly grab hold of the Kegel while throwing and catching a ball, jumping, and forcefully pushing a ball into a table. The quick grasp of the contraction can train the muscles to counter quickly approaching forces. I call this agility training for the pelvic floor. Brute force is important, however, quick reaction timing of that forceful pelvic floor contraction is paramount to continent success!

Teaching a patient's pelvic floor to react quickly to an unexpected change in position, a stumble, or an unexpected jolt to the abdomen is a great way to train automaticity. Having a patient hold a ball and resist changing pressures on the ball while her eyes are closed can create such a simulation. Setting up a training circuit and having the patient literally and figuratively bounce quickly from one station to the next can also gradually train the patient to automatically Kegel with a novel activity and with a rapid change in position.

Sitting and standing on uneven surfaces such as a therapy ball or a half ball (Bosu, en Francais) can help create lifelike scenarios that challenge the pelvic floor. While on these surfaces, I ask the patient to attempt to hold a Kegel while the trunk and lower extremity muscles quickly engage to keep balance. With these simulations, the pelvic floor can learn to respond to sudden forces that positional changes may apply to the abdominal and pelvic cavities. This quick response training helps to improve the automaticity of the pelvic floor's contraction. Progressing to walking on uneven surfaces while Kegeling can prepare the patient for traversing uneven ground as when trail running, hiking, or walking across a construction site whereby the body may shift positions unexpectedly. Uneven surface negotiation can thusly combine strength, endurance, timing, and agility, while putting the Kegel into functional practice.

Holding a Kegel against multiple bouts of pressure can improve the endurance of the pelvic floor muscles. The successive changes in intra-abdominal pressure can resemble real life scenarios involving a multitude of steps, a series of sneezes, and a hearty bout of laughter. Progressing still, I ask patients while biking or walking to moderately Kegel for 10 seconds, and then add a burst of an extra strong contraction before releasing. This long hold followed by a burst of a finale can help patients prepare for a scenario of walking up steps and suddenly coughing, or jogging along a familiar route and throwing a high-five to an oncoming runner. Endurance to sustain a moderate contraction and readiness to strongly hold can prepare patients for life's rigorous activities and unexpected jolts.

Preparing a patient for life's unexpected surprises by simulating activities requiring altered levels of holding power can help prepare her for the activities that invoke the most incontinence. Asking the patient to practice the moderate hold followed by a more firmly held contraction when returning a tennis serve, kicking a soccer ball, or a blocking a basketball shot can be an excellent way to exercise the pelvic floor and give the patient a way to incorporate Kegels into an athletic part of her day. When the patient notices she is automatically contracting the pelvic floor with her activities, full independence is near.

The more quickly patients can time the Kegel around an activity and the more complicated the activity, the greater the automaticity of the Kegel's response to intra-abdominal pressures in daily life. Holding the contraction throughout one activity, then changing to a different activity can create carryover of the contraction into novel tasks. In the clinic, we may not be able to simulate every single circumstance patients encounter over the course of their lives. However, we can instill the notion that it may be necessary to contract in order to counter the forces brought about by all rigorous activities. Ideally, patients' *home exercise programs* transform into *life exercise programs*. Such a transformation usually develops gradually as I encourage the patients to Kegel around more and more of their days' activities. Soon the *exercises* can become *automatic responses* that counter life's intra-abdominal pressures.

It is important to note that patients may find it a daunting task, if not impossible, to Kegel with all of their daily activities. This is particularly the case for patients who have severe cases of stress urinary incontinence, whereby just Kegeling for three seconds three times consecutively is a huge feat. Setting short term goals too high may set incontinence rehabilitation up for failure. Therefore, I would recommend starting slowly and helping the patient to realize that the effort to contract the pelvic floor will ease and the length of the contractions will grow.

Once the isolated contraction is achieved, the ease of timing around and during an activity will likely build. As part of her independent exercise program, I may recommend having the patient start with a sit to stand transfer. This is a task in daily life that is premeditated, versus a sneeze that may sneak up out of the blue. The patient would have time to concentrate on Kegeling before standing from a dinner chair, before getting out of her vehicle, or before getting out of bed. Supplying a specific activity for the patient to independently Kegel around is usually a more successful approach to a home program than telling the patient that the Kegel needs to occur with all activities from the get-go.

My quickest roads to recovery, therefore, usually start with a suggestion of just one or two tasks around which to Kegel. To progress, I gradually add more activities to the mix, one at a time. Oftentimes, patients take it upon themselves to progressively add more tasks around which to Kegel, eventually realizing they can easily contract with activities periodically throughout their day. At this point, a home exercise program is no longer a set amount of exercises. Kegeling starts to envelope daily living tasks and the exercises no longer usurp precious time from an already busy schedule. Kegeling around a growing number of activities can help to fully integrate the pelvic floor's hold and resolve stress urinary incontinence with life's daily pursuits.

Figure 14 is an example of an exercise sheet I give to patients for practicing the almighty, isolated Kegel. The tricks I use to cue the correct muscles are explained. The long and short holds are emphasized, and the timing of such contractions is explicit.

Figure 14. A home exercise program for pelvic floor muscle training.

Pelvic Floor Exercises
Page 1

Kegeling: Contracting the pelvic floor muscles.

- *Attempt to stop the urine stream once per week. Simulate stopping the urine stream to further practice.*
    - Try to stop the flow of urine once you have started to void, but only once per week. Stopping the urine stream contracts the pelvic floor muscles, which are used to Kegel.
    - While contracting the pelvic floor (Kegeling), you should feel the pelvic floor being pulled toward your chest, drawn further into your body (upward if you are sitting or standing).
    - Continue practicing with a voiding simulation, contracting the same muscles that would stop the urine stream if you were voiding. This can and should be done to improve the strength of the pelvic floor muscles, but not while actually urinating more than once per week.
- *Tampon trick*:
    - Insert a tampon halfway into your vagina (with clean hands).
    - Use the muscles surrounding the tampon (the pelvic floor muscles) to pull the tampon upward, further into the vagina. This muscle contraction is the Kegel.
    - To progress, gently pull on the tampon string with your fingers. Contract the pelvic floor muscles to resist the tugging on the tampon.
- *Pillow trick*:
    - Sitting on a soft pillow or contoured cushion, note the pressure against the perineum or undersurface of the pelvic floor.
    - Contract the pelvic floor muscles (Kegel).
    - With the Kegel, there should be a lifting sensation whereby less pressure is felt against the perineum or undersurface of the pelvic floor.

Pelvic Floor Exercises
Page 2

Sustained Kegels: Long pelvic floor muscle contractions for endurance training.

- Contract the pelvic floor muscles (Kegel) for 10 seconds, relax for 10-20 seconds.
- Repeat 10-second holds 10 times, 3-10 sets per day.

Quick Kegels: To learn to quickly contract and relax the pelvic floor muscles for agility and added bursts of strength.

- Contract the pelvic floor muscles (Kegel) as quickly as you can, contracting only as long as needed to find the muscles and only as firmly as you can in isolation. Preferable contractions are 2 seconds or less, resting for 2-4 seconds between each contraction.
- Repeat 10 quick contractions 10 times, 3-10 sets per day.

Timing: Hold the contraction *around* an activity, starting the contraction before the activity, holding during the activity and only releasing after the activity is complete.

- Contract the pelvic floor (Kegel) *around* a cough or sneeze.
- Contract the pelvic floor (Kegel) *around* transferring from sit to stand.
- Gradually add activities around which to Kegel, for example lifting an object and stepping up and down a step.

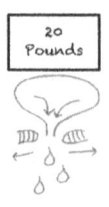

Too Much Too Fast Is NOT Recommended

Overworking the pelvic floor muscles can lead to a temporary regression. Such overexertion can disrupt the ability to contract against intra-abdominal pressure and lead to incontinent episodes. We want to expedite care, however, too much too soon is detrimental to progress. It is important that clinicians ask patients how they respond to the level and vigor of the treatment sessions and home exercises. Patients should communicate whether they improve or worsen after each treatment and with the home exercises. The same level of activity across two sessions may have different effects depending on the cumulative effects of the exercises. Adequate recovery time is necessary to strengthen the pelvic floor.

Overly exerting the pelvic floor muscles is similar to running multiple marathons. A marathon, for most people, is not a feasible task to repeat multiple days in a row. Eventually the marathons can lead to an accumulation of physical stress that disallows taking another effective step. Kegeling can have a similar cumulative effect. In cases of an overly exerted pelvic floor, the end result can be an unfortunate incontinent episode. Treatments should be adjusted to prevent overexertion. To exemplify, if a patient is planning to implement the Kegel while performing a rigorous task later in the day after a treatment session, or has just completed such, I adjust the amount of force and length of Kegel holds in the treatment session. The home program and treatment sessions should complement one another, not figuratively run the pelvic floor into the ground.

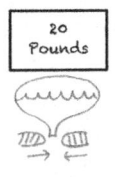

Acquiring a Resting Tone in the Pelvic Floor Muscles

A result I seek in training the pelvic floor musculature is a moderate resting tone that does not require conscious concentration. This is a very important statement to make to patients who cannot fathom fully contracting the pelvic floor constantly. Just as a flaccid or weak quadriceps (thigh) muscle needs exercise to acquire a moderate tone to hold a person in standing, the pelvic floor needs exercise to build a resting tone to hold against urine flow. Normally we do not consciously think about the tone that is established in our quadriceps while standing on our feet, but we are certainly aware of the quadriceps when we are climbing a large step, or squatting and lifting a heavy box. Eventually, patients should not even have to think about holding a resting tone in the pelvic floor. A solid resting tone should emerge and when extra force is needed to fend off abrupt or sustained increases in intra-abdominal pressure, the pelvic floor should be ready to deliver.

We have now come full circle with the training of the pelvic floor's contraction against stress urinary incontinence. The patients should find the muscles, isolate the muscles, apply the contractions around and during activities, gradually build a resting tone, and maintain a healthy resting tone by continuing to Kegel with daily activities. Stronger and more agile contractions can occur as patients contract to counter increasing magnitudes of intra-abdominal pressure and improve the reaction timing against unforeseen pulses of intra-abdominal force. Finally, carrying over the contraction into novel activities for full functional integration can bring patients back to a life without the fear of incontinence.

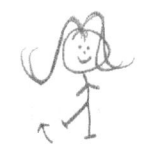

Patients with Stress Urinary Incontinence Trudged into My Care, but with Rehabilitation, They Danced Out

To exemplify my treatment scenarios, let me introduce a few patients that achieved continence with a progression of Kegel implementations. Although stress urinary incontinence was the consistent medical diagnosis, each individual patient was distinct and treated based on individual needs. In each case, remedying the underlying cause and building strength and agility in the pelvic floor muscles were keys to regaining continence. Continence with all activity, regardless of bodily position, activity rigor, and level of fatigue, was and continues to be the universal goal of stress urinary incontinence rehabilitation. Similarities may abound in each case, but it is important to see each patient as an individual with specific needs and specific goals.

Weakness Stemming from Disuse

Incontinence can arise out of pelvic floor muscle weakness simply due to lack of contraction. This was the case for a woman named Jenna who could not Kegel voluntarily without the incorporation of her abdominals. She could not stop the flow of urine, even though she did not have confounding factors of neural damage or malalignment of the pelvis. Jenna was a case of weakness due to disuse. Having had two children, the length-tension relationship of her pelvic floor muscles may have been disadvantageously lengthened due overstretching with childbirth. Having neglected her pelvic floor muscles after childbirth, her pre-childbirth strength had started to dwindle.

    Jenna was moderately high functioning with respect to continence, but did present with some pelvic floor weakness, which lead to leaking with rigorous activity. She was able to hold while walking and with a single sit to stand transfer. She was not, however, able to hold throughout the bout of sneezes she regularly experienced with allergies. She was also not able to counter repeated pressures whilst climbing a flight of 12 stairs in her home. Add carrying a heavy object up the stairs, like a full suitcase, and she was unable to hold against the abdominal pressure even stepping up one stair. The cumulative effect of repeated pressures in the abdominal region fatigued the pelvic floor to a point of failure and incontinence was had.

    The scenarios that lead to Jenna's pelvic floor muscle failure were dissected and used in her treatments to achieve successful continence. First, I asked Jenna to contract the pelvic floor repeatedly in sitting, standing, and lying supine to allow her to become confident with an isolated hold. With a successfully isolated contraction checked off the list, she started contracting before and while stepping up a stair, and then releasing. She would then contract once again before and while stepping down. When Kegeling around ascending and descending a stair became a nonissue, she then stepped up and down multiple steps, all the while holding the pelvic floor in a contracted state. In time, Jenna was able to hold a Kegel while repeatedly ascending and descending stairs. Once this was accomplished, she learned to Kegel moderately and to add a strong burst every three steps. The added burst of muscle contraction prepared her for countering the unexpected increases in abdominal pressure that would occur with a sneeze when her allergies arose.

Next, Jenna progressively carried heavier and heavier weights up the step with the Kegel timing intact. She started carrying a five-pound weight up one step, then up two steps, and then up three steps. She would hold with a moderate amount of force and add a strong burst every three steps, in case a sneeze would arrive. We progressed the weight and length of holds, adding appropriate rest breaks so as to not over-fatigue the pelvic floor muscles. Practicing the moderate Kegel with added bursts of strong holds paved the way to Jenna's successful continence. In time, climbing stairs with a suitcase in hand and a sneeze on the brink was countered with a strong pelvic floor ready to combat any thought of incontinence.

Targeting the Activities Most Important to the Patient First:

Timing, Interval Training, and Kicking the Kegel into Gear

A sense of motivation is heightened when a patient is in control of the rehabilitative activities. I have found that patient-guided treatments accomplish the ultimate goal of continence with all activity. They can help patients overcome the specific challenges that are most problematic and most likely to cause their incontinence. If a patient has a strong desire to run, perform Tae Kwon

Do, and jump on a trampoline with her children, the exercises should be geared toward those passions, all the while guiding the patient with pacing strategies so as to not over-fatigue the pelvic floor. Helping a patient to resume her passions can get her back to 'living' and bring her an air of relief. Strenuous activity is a means of stress release. Giving a patient her passions back one or two at a time can help her to see the proverbial light. The stage is then set for even greater motivation to fully achieve continence with all activities including her passions, regardless of their demand on the pelvic floor.

To accomplish the reintroduction of a strenuous activity into a patient's life, I find it helpful to suggest performing that activity at the time of day when the pelvic floor is most up for the challenge. If a patient has the liberty to change her schedule, it would be best to perform the strenuous activity early in the day, before the pelvic floor muscles are fatigued from a hard day's work. Helping a patient strategize a change in schedule is integral in helping her to achieve her chief goal early on in the rehabilitation process. Changing a schedule can be a daunting task. With the motivation to resume her favorite daily activity, however, the change may come more readily and soon she will have achieved continence with one of her most important activities.

To help a patient resume her rigorous activity, I ask her to perform *interval training* for the pelvic floor muscles. To use running as an example, I will often start the patient with walking even just one step while Kegeling. Kegeling around one step at a time can then progress to Kegeling around multiple steps as appropriate for the patient's level of ability and, of course, fatigue. The next step in training would be Kegeling around a small jump. Kegeling around one small jump, then around multiple jumps can eventually pave the way for a successful Kegel when running. Kegeling around jumping on both feet with the feet together, then with the feet apart, and then Kegeling around jumping on one foot would be the next successive hurdles. Once the pelvic floor's contraction can withstand multiple jumps, Kegeling around intervals of running may ensue. It may sound like a long ways away from running, but the association of Kegeling with each small step can lay the groundwork for the grand finale.

Interval training worked wonders for Kristen, an avid runner who, after having a child, could not run without incontinence. Kristen's muscles had become weak and could not stand up to the intra-abdominal forces that running applied to her bladder. Once she was able to Kegel successfully around repeated jumps, she started Kegeling with an interval running program. One minute of running, two minutes of walking, one minute of rest repeated three times gradually regained Kristen a dry run! Integrating small bouts of Kegels into a gradually progressed running regime regained Kristen continence while out on the road.

Some runners with incontinence have not necessarily lost the ability to automatically Kegel with all strenuous activity, but they have misplaced the ability to do so with repeated jolts. An example of such an individual is Julie. Julie had no incontinent episodes when lifting her ever-growing six month-old baby, standing from sitting, coughing, walking, and stepping up stairs. Running, though, was her incontinence instigator. We found that a round of consciously Kegeling was needed before tackling the run. Why wouldn't her automatic contractions with lifting, walking, or stair climbing be enough of a warm-up? Because she did not have to *think* about Kegeling with those activities. Julie needed assistance with timing the pelvic floor to contract around *a specific activity*, not just to contract. In this case, a warm-up of *conscious Kegels* was needed before attempting to Kegel with the strenuous task of running. Adding five minutes of Kegels, during which Julie actively contracted the pelvic floor muscles with the contraction on the forefront of her mind, allowed her to run for ten minutes in the clinic. How did Julie add the warm-up to an already busy day? By *consciously Kegeling* with her morning routine of lifting her baby repeatedly, while making her bed, or while preparing her lunch for her workday. After the warm-up of conscious Kegels, Julie was able to Kegel around run/walk/rest intervals and progress to her beloved 30-minute hard run before the start her long work day.

As exemplified by the previous two cases, patients with the same diagnosis should be treated as individuals. Despite Julie and Kristen having the same diagnosis of stress urinary incontinence with the chief problem being incontinence with running, each was treated a bit differently. Kristen needed interval training due to sheer muscle weakness. Julie's muscles were not weak; she needed a boost of conscious Kegeling to kick them into gear to specifically combat the repeated jolt of running. Similar training methods are often used for multiple patients, but in conjunction with specific techniques targeting the distinctive roots of each patient's individual problem.

Several of my patients had come to physical therapy seeking continence with jumping and kicking in order to resume kickboxing and Tae Kwon Do. Both are forms of incredible exercise, self-defense, and stress release. Without such exercise and release, a long day can feel even longer. But, a bout of frustrating incontinence can pounce with an attempt to jump or to kick. When her favorite activity requires both, a patient with incontinence can feel hopeless. Jumping can add an incredible amount of intra-abdominal pressure and kicking opens the legs potentiating a disadvantageous lengthening of the pelvic floor muscle fibers. It is important to listen to the patient's description of when incontinence occurs. Do the incontinent episodes occur with all of her jumping and kicking attempts? Do they occur at the beginning of a session? At the end? For some, the pelvic floor contraction is strong enough to combat incontinence for a short while, but fatigue sets in and a full session of kickboxing or Tae Kwon Do is not possible without an incontinent episode. For others, incontinence occurs with any and all of the kickboxing and Tae Kwon Do maneuvers. For both ends of the spectrum and all cases in between, a detailed series of treatments can spring the patients back in action.

    At the outset of therapy, Jessica was not able to Kegel with any of her Tae Kwon Do maneuvers for any length of time. Her rehabilitation commenced with instruction to contract around simple, less strenuous tasks to introduce the idea of timing the Kegel around an activity. We progressed from Kegeling around one small, slow kick at a time, to Kegeling around multiple small kicks, then to Kegeling around one large kick, and finally to Kegeling around repeated large kicks. With a concentrated effort to Kegel around each kick or series of kicks, a resting tone was achieved and her automatic contraction halted further incontinent episodes. A similar progression with jumping ensued. Starting with a combination of small jumps with kicks, Jessica progressed to large jumps with kicks, and then to a full hour of Tae Kwon Do without a drop of incontinence.

My patients have often expressed deep gratitude for helping them take back a key life event that had been stolen by incontinence. Even if a patient has an incontinent episode lifting a heavy box at the end of the day due to pelvic floor muscle fatigue, she is often ecstatic to have been able to run 30 minutes the morning prior. The end result is for the patient to be able to lift that box despite the day's activities. But while building endurance for complete continence, I recommend focusing on the patient's top priorities first. Overcoming the incontinence that occurs with the activities the patient deems most important can give the patient power. This power can motivate the patient to continue to build endurance to achieve continence with whatever life throws her way.

Catching Stress Urinary Incontinence Early... Or, Even by Chance

For justification of treatment, cases of stress urinary incontinence do *not* have to be so severe that leakage occurs with every activity. On the contrary, I highly recommend treating before the leaking becomes the norm. Early intervention can reduce the amount of time it takes to train the pelvic floor to counter the forces associated with life's affected activities. I have found that early intervention leads to faster results, seeing as the patients are starting out with a higher level of functional pelvic floor contraction. (This is similar to early intervention for several other conditions like imbalance, back pain, and muscle strains.) The patients starting therapy early are often able to perform a Kegel with moderate activity, and total control has not been lost. Oftentimes, patients can resume all activity incontinence-free in a relatively short period of time. Catching the incontinence early can allow patients to rehabilitate as quickly as with one visit!

A glaring example of how early intervention is remarkably effective walked into my office with the fear that she would someday lose control of her bladder to the point of requiring surgical intervention. With the assistance of a chair's counter-pressure holding the weight of the pelvic floor contents in check, Linda was able to hold against a sneeze and a cough while seated. However, she was unable to hold her pelvic floor muscles with sneezing and coughing while in a standing position. Linda noted incontinence when transferring from standing to sitting and with stepping up and down a step. She was able to hold without movement in sitting, standing, and lying supine. But, her muscles fatigued after holding for only 3-4 seconds, and she was unable to isolate the pelvic floor contraction from the gluteal (buttocks) muscles. Although Linda had some control over the pelvic floor, it was not enough to counter moderate to heavy exertion. (See Figure 15.)

Linda's first task was to isolate the pelvic floor contraction from the gluteals (buttocks muscles), then timing the Kegels successfully around activities could ensue. At her first visit, Linda learned to appropriately isolate the pelvic floor muscles. I advised her contract the pelvic floor in isolation even if the force of this isolated contraction was merely half of that generated when co-contracting the gluteals (buttocks). Learning to isolate the pelvic floor was integral, but timing the contraction around the activities that caused incontinence was needed to make the Kegel functional. With the isolated Kegel in check, Linda learned to contract before the start of a transfer, before a bout of sneezes, and before taking a step. Linda learned to hold during the activity, and to release only after the activities' completion. After this one training session, Linda practiced her isolated contraction and began to add Kegels around her daily activities. From a co-contraction of the gluteals (buttocks), to successful isolation, to timing integration, Linda returned a week later having resumed her active daily life without incontinence.

Yes, Linda's success occurred after one visit and a week of training. Once a patient achieves isolation of the pelvic floor muscle contraction, strength and endurance can be built correctly. Continence can then be seen on the horizon. By learning to start the contraction before an activity, hold the contraction during the activity, and release only after completing the activity, continence can be achieved! Catching the incontinence at early stages can therefore make the trip to recovery a quick one!

Figure 15: An initial evaluation of a patient with early stages of stress urinary incontinence:

Diagnosis: Stress urinary incontinence

Upon evaluation, the following were noted:
1. Patient reports abrupt onset of stress urinary incontinence ~ 8/1/13.
2. Patient noted incontinent episodes with coughing initially, then noted episodes with sneezing, stepping up a step, and otherwise applying intra-abdominal pressure.
3. Patient is not able to isolate the pelvic floor from gluteals. She reports ability to stop the urine stream and is able to hold pelvic floor for 3-4 seconds in standing.
4. Patient is able to counter strong intra-abdominal pressures while sitting.
5. However, in standing, patient is unable to counter the heavy, abrupt, forceful intra-abdominal pressure sustained with a sneeze or cough.
6. With walking, stepping up a step, and sitting from standing, patient is unable to hold.
7. Therefore, the missing link appears to be the ability to hold a strong Kegel contraction against added pressure in standing, without a chair to provide the counter-pressure to support the pelvic floor.
8. Strengthening in standing will ensue.
9. Contraction timing will be enforced to regain the Kegel's automatic contraction against forceful surges of intra-abdominal pressure in standing and whilst moving about on foot.
10. Should electrical stimulation or electrical biofeedback be appropriate, measures will be taken.

Plan/Goals:
1. Independent with home exercise program.
2. Pelvic floor muscle contraction isolated.
3. Independent timing of pelvic floor hold for countering incontinence.
4. No episodes of incontinence with coughing or sneezing in standing.
5. No episodes of incontinence with all activity.

"Aha!! I haven't used those muscles since my husband passed away 10 years ago!"

Catching a patient's condition of stress urinary incontinence may happen by chance. A patient may be referred to physical therapy for a back strain, and with either a line of questioning or with the introduction to Kegeling as a means of core control, incontinence can be unveiled. This was the case for Leilani, a patient who came in to see me with a low back strain after a motor vehicle accident. I introduced her to core exercises as a means of lumbar stabilization, including the Kegel exercise to contract the pelvic floor. She was having a difficult time Kegeling. I asked her to simulate stopping the flow of urine and she whispered in my ear, "I can't"! Leilani then reported that she had developed stress urinary incontinence years before the motor vehicle accident. She reportedly could not find the pelvic floor muscles. Low back and pelvic injury can be a source of bowel and bladder problems, as can inadequate pelvic floor exercise. In this case, Leilani had not voluntarily and consciously contracted the pelvic floor muscles "in years"!!! And, automatic contractions had not been enough to sustain strength in her pelvic floor muscles. In one treatment with electrical vaginal stimulation, she joyfully yelped, "Aha!! I haven't used those muscles since my husband passed away 10 years ago!" After that one session, Leilani was able to find the pelvic floor muscles independently and practice contracting her way to continence, and core stabilization!

Tackling Stress Urinary Incontinence In a Bit More Detail

Direct physical trauma to the vaginal walls, the pelvic floor, and the lumbar-pelvic (low back and pelvic) region can lead to a difficult recovery of the pelvic floor muscles. With such trauma, the pelvic floor muscles may *turn off*. It is our job to *turn them back on*. Before a trauma, the pelvic floor not only may contract automatically to close the external sphincter, it may also contract to hold the lumbar-pelvic (low back and pelvic) region intact. After the trauma, consciously Kegeling may be needed in order to help stabilize the spine. Because of the pelvic floor's dual function of stabilization and continence control, incontinence resolution is often also on the rehabilitation agenda.

As previously mentioned, malalignment of the pelvis and sacrum can lead to *and* stem from pelvic floor weakness. This weakness in turn can lead to numerous cases of stress urinary incontinence. A very common scenario tied to stress urinary incontinence is the elevation of one ilium (side of the pelvis) in relation to the other. (See previous Figure 8.) How do I tackle incontinence, warranting pelvic floor *isolation*, intertwined with pelvic asymmetries needing a *co-contraction* of the pelvic floor and the abdominals for stabilization? By correcting the elevation with manual distraction of the limb on the elevated side, teaching self-correction stretches for home, ensuring isolated pelvic floor contraction to counter the incontinence, then adding full core exercises (contracting the pelvic floor, gently pulling the navel to the spine to contract the deep abdominal muscles, and breathing through the diaphragm) to stabilize the pelvic region after isolation of the pelvic floor muscles is achieved. (See Figures 16a and 16b.)

Figure 16a. An illustration depicting a self-help correction of an elevated ilium (side of pelvis) (left). A family member assisting in elevation correction (right.)

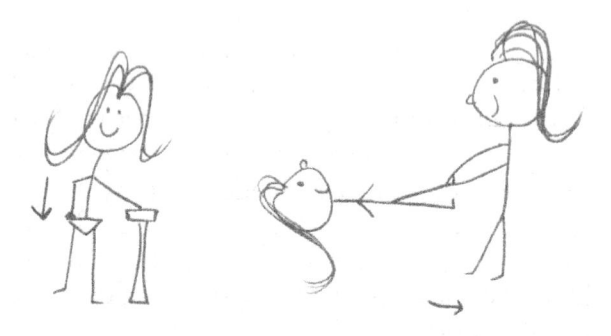

Figure 16b. An illustration of a self-help stretch.

To correct a right-sided elevation, the patient stretches the right side of the low back. The patient is to lunge with the left foot in front of the right, lean onto the left hand on a supported surface, and reach with the right hand forward and to the left for 10-20 seconds. When finished stretching, the patient is to use the left hand to push herself upright.

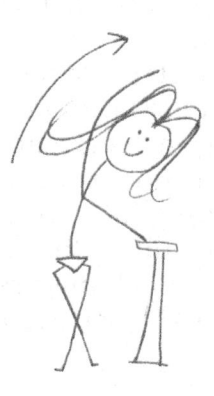

Clinicians, while distracting the limb, ask the patient to contract her pelvic floor muscles with a Kegel exercise. If the asymmetry is indeed contributing to difficulty with Kegeling, the patient should find it easier to Kegel while her limb is gently pulled and her pelvis is realigned into symmetry. This distraction can pull the ilium (side of pelvis) into alignment, thereby placing the pelvic floor muscle fibers in a more favorable length-tension relationship. This alignment, therefore, can improve the pelvic floor muscles' contractile force. As previously stated, once the patient is able to isolate the pelvic floor muscles, adding core exercises incorporating contractions of the pelvic floor and the deep abdominals can better keep the pelvis in alignment.

Even when contracting the pelvic floor and abdominal muscles together for the core contraction, it is important to isolate the pelvic floor first, then add the abdominals. This order of business can help to reinforce the pelvic floor isolation when the isolation is needed to hold urine flow. Clinicians, it is important to educate the patient on the proper timing of the pelvic floor and abdominal contractions and how they interfere and interact with one another.

In cases whereby the pelvic floor training is needed in isolation to counter incontinence and in conjunction with the abdominals to support the core, I often tell the patient that she is working on two separate conditions, each needing different exercises. I often say, "Everything is connected and needs to be treated as such. But in this case, think of yourself as two separate patients to keep from confusing the pelvic floor." I find that by telling the patient in this scenario to think of herself as two patients, she is better able to grasp when to isolate and when to co-contract. As the automaticity of the urinary control improves, the patient should be able to isolate when controlling urination, and co-contract to keep the pelvis aligned without confusion.

Elevation of one side of the pelvis often recurs with the application of body weight through the limb on the same side as the elevation. Stepping up a step, walking, running, hiking, and lunging onto the affected side add pressure through the limb, and this unilateral (one-sided) pressure can shift the pelvis out of alignment. The repeated self-help stretches can remedy the shift, and core exercises 10 seconds 10 times per day can help keep the shift from recurring. As with the pelvic floor in isolation, strengthening and timing of the core may take practice. The stretches can help to remedy the shift until the core is strong enough to hold the pelvis in place. (See previous Figures 16a and 16b.)

In the early stages of therapy, I ask the patient contract only the pelvic floor with these unilateral activities. Why not engage the full core right away? Because the intra-abdominal pressure they incur on the bladder can cause incontinence. The pelvic floor being part of the core can partially help to stabilize the ilia (sides of pelvis) to keep them from shifting to a greater degree. When the isolation of the pelvic floor becomes automatic for urinary control I ask the patient to then add the full core's co-contraction of the abdominals and the pelvic floor muscles *around* these activities to firmly stabilize the pelvic joints against the shift...but only when the patient is not trying to counter a full bladder! Struggling to hold back urine flow with a *very* full bladder can happen whether we regularly experience incontinence or not. Everyone's muscles have their breaking point! At these times, I have the patient revert to holding only the pelvic floor, especially when she may be running to the restroom! To reinforce urinary control and joint alignment, I recommend that the patient perform Kegels in isolation and full core exercises as separate entities. I help the patient figure the times when she can integrate the exercises consciously into her day. After a stretch to reinforce the alignment, and without having an urge to urinate, the patient can perform the core exercises (Kegel plus abdominal contraction) with walking about or going up and down the stairs. With the activities that do not firmly press on one limb at a time, like when transferring from sitting to standing with equal pressure through both feet, I recommend isolating the Kegel as the conscious exercise. The isolated Kegel and the full core contractions will likely become automatic, but it is important to separate the two initially, and *consciously* perform each in order to teach appropriate timing.

    Molly presented with stress urinary incontinence and ilial asymmetry in need of correction and stabilization. Her right lumbar paraspinals (low back muscles) were very tense and restricted. The muscle tension was consistent with her habitual standing posture, which elevated the right side of her pelvis. Reducing the tension in her lumbar paraspinals
(low back muscles) and distracting the right limb gained Molly ilial (pelvic) symmetry and greater ease with pelvic floor contractions. (See previous Figure 16a.) But, incontinence training and pelvic stabilization as described above were needed for Molly to fully rehabilitate. (See Figure 17.)

Figure 17. An initial evaluation of a patient experiencing stress urinary incontinence with moderate to strenuous activity, and presenting with asymmetrical pelvic alignment.

Diagnoses: Stress urinary incontinence with right ilial elevation

Upon evaluation, the following were noted:
1. Patient reports stress urinary incontinence with jumping jacks, jumping on a trampoline, and running. The onset of incontinence reportedly occurred upon resuming exercise ~ 10/25/13.
2. Right ilial elevation is noted with pain radiating from the piriformis region to the medial and posterior thigh (buttocks to inner and back side of thigh) on the right.
3. Tension in the lumbar paraspinals is greater on the right versus left, correlating with an upward pull on the right ilium.
4. With a right ilial distraction stretch, patient held a stronger pelvic floor contraction. This suggests that ilial obliquities contribute at least partially to her difficulty contracting the pelvic floor muscles.
5. Ilial asymmetry likely disadvantageously lengthens the pelvic floor muscle fibers weakening their contractile strength.
6. Ilial asymmetry may disrupt the neural pathways with foraminal encroachment. Irritation of the nerves may weaken the pelvic floor muscles and contribute to pain.
7. A complication presents with the need for full core stabilization to hold ilial symmetry to afford a most proficient pelvic floor contraction. The full core contraction includes activation of the transverse abdominis. Such a contraction, though, increases intra-abdominal pressure and can enhance the incontinence.
8. Patient does report contracting the pelvic floor as an exercise, however, upon examination of such, she is doing so in conjunction with a strong abdominal hold.
9. The patient's abdominal contraction leads to increased intra-abdominal pressure, which appears to make countering urine flow even more difficult. Therefore, the patient's own attempts at pelvic floor exercises likely perpetuate and worsen the incontinence.
10. Given the onset of incontinence in conjunction with resuming running and jumping, the pelvic floor is likely not adequately conditioned to counter the inherent intra-abdominal pressure with such exercise.
11. Running adds asymmetrical pressure across the pelvic joints. The ensuing malalignment, in turn, likely hinders a strong pelvic floor

contraction.
12. We have commenced treatment with ilial distraction to align the pelvis, and with isolating the pelvic floor contraction to counter incontinence and provide partial stabilization of the pelvic joints.
13. Once the isolated pelvic floor contraction is mastered, we will then add the transverse abdominis contraction to better hold the pelvis in alignment. This improved alignment is expected to improve the strength of the isolated pelvic floor contraction and reduce pain.
14. Should electrical stimulation and/or electrical biofeedback be appropriate and necessary, measures will be taken.

Plan/Goals:
1. Independent with HEP—ongoing.
2. Pelvic floor muscle contraction isolated.
3. Independent isolation and timing of pelvic floor for countering incontinence.
4. Contraction of the full core for pelvic stabilization with the understanding of when to contract the pelvic floor in isolation for urinary control.
5. No episodes of incontinence with running, jumping or other activity.

◆

Emma presented with stress urinary incontinence in conjunction with pelvic asymmetries as well. She had difficulty isolating the pelvic floor from the abdominals and had difficulty commencing a contraction of the pelvic floor quickly. Her right ilium (side of pelvis) was elevated, and she admitted to carrying both of her children on the right side of her pelvis with her pelvis tilted upwards on the right. (See previous Figure 8). This carrying method was the likely instigator of the elevation of the right side of her pelvis. Why did the incontinence occur after the birth of the second and not the first child? Quite possibly due to an accumulation of physical stress inherent in carrying two children, or one child at a time twice as often. The elevated positioning likely pulled the pelvic floor muscle fibers into a disadvantageously lengthened position, and the physical stress of carrying and lifting two children likely fatigued the pelvic floor, leading to incontinence. (See Figure 18.)

Figure 18. An initial evaluation of a patient with stress urinary incontinence after the birth of her second child.

Diagnoses: Stress urinary incontinence with right ilial elevation

Upon evaluation, the following were noted:

1. Patient reports onset of stress urinary incontinence ~ 1/11/13 after the birth of her second child. Patient notes particular difficulty holding urine when passing gas.
2. Patient has difficulty quickly contracting and holding the pelvic floor contracted in isolation of the abdominal musculature.
3. The stronger the patient attempts to contract the pelvic floor the greater the abdominal engagement. The co-contraction is counterproductive to holding continent.
4. Right ilial elevation is consistent with holding her children on the right side of her pelvis and with greater tension in right versus left lumbar paraspinals.
5. With correction of elevation, patient is able to isolate the pelvic floor contraction.
6. A complication presents with the need for core stabilization to hold ilial symmetry to afford the most proficient pelvic floor contraction. The full core contraction includes activation of the transverse abdominis. Such a contraction increases intra-abdominal pressure, which can enhance the incontinence.
7. Once patient is able to integrate isolation of the pelvic floor into daily activities, we will commence full core contraction so as to hold the pelvis in alignment.
8. Should electrical stimulation and/or electrical biofeedback be appropriate and necessary, measures will be taken.

Plan/Goals:

1. Independent with home exercise program.

2. Pelvic floor muscle contraction isolated.
3. Independent timing of pelvic floor hold for countering incontinence.
4. Ilial symmetry held with home exercise program only.
5. Contraction of full core for pelvic stabilization with the understanding of when to contract pelvic floor for urinary control and when to contract the core for pelvic stabilization.
6. No episodes of incontinence.

◆ ◆ ◆

Emma's treatment encompassed correction of the ilial asymmetries, strength and agility training, and eventual incorporation of the full core. With treatment to release the tension of the right lumbar paraspinals (low back muscles), the ilia (sides of pelvis) were aligned. With such alignment, she was able to contract the pelvic floor in isolation of the abdominals, and was able to eventually time the Kegel around excessive bouts of added intra-abdominal pressure. In Emma's case, it appeared as though the agility of quickly contracting in isolation after passing gas was integral to remaining dry. Her actual strength improved rather quickly, but the quick bursts of isolated contraction were the missing link. Her attempted quick bursts of pelvic floor contraction incorporated contraction of the abdominal muscles. The resulting increase in intra-abdominal pressure further pressed on the bladder making it more difficult to hold her urine. The isolated quick burst was gained with timing around a series of quick presses on a therapy ball, tossing and catching a 4-pound medicine ball, as well as timing around simulations of passing gas. Once the isolated contraction was second nature, full core exercises were introduced to hold the pelvis in alignment. In the meantime, to complement her treatment of the pelvis, Emma stretched the right side of her low back diligently and refrained from carrying her children on a raised ilium (side of pelvis). Eventually, Emma's pelvis stayed aligned and she was able to integrate isolated contractions into activities of daily living, freeing herself from incontinence.

In another case whereby incontinence occurred with passing gas, gaining the ability to contract the front portion of the pelvic floor while releasing the rear portion was key. Alexis was unable to control the urinary flow when she passed gas, but was able to hold in most other scenarios. Why? Because although the normal contraction sequence when engaging the pelvic floor is to contract the rear portion first, then the front, there are times when the front portion must contract while the rear remains relaxed, as when passing gas with a rather full bladder. Alexis's treatment was challenging due to her need to take her conscious contraction one step further. To practice, I recommended Alexis sit on a cushioned chair with extra pressure at the anterior aspect (front) of the pelvic floor. This pressure at the front end allowed her to feel where she was to contract specifically to hold her urine when she needed to pass gas. The chair acted as a tactile (or touch) cue to assist Alexis in knowing when she was contracting and releasing the front portion of the pelvic floor. Alexis practiced relaxing the pelvic floor, but instead of first releasing the front portion and then releasing the backside, she had to release only the backside. It was not an easy task, but the tactile cuing assisted Alexis in achieving the necessary muscle control. Alexis also practiced quick Kegels like Emma did in order to gain agility in the pelvic floor muscles. This allowed for a quick hold of the entire pelvic floor in case the front portion of the pelvic floor failed. In approximately three weeks, Alexis was able to pass gas without incontinence.

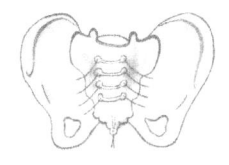

Weakened Abdominal Musculature and a Tie to Stress Urinary Incontinence

Is this a paradox?

Another factor that may potentiate stress urinary incontinence is a weak transverse abdominis muscle. Yes, I am speculating that a *weakened deep abdominal muscle* may indirectly lead to incontinence. How is this possible when the pelvic floor fights to counter abdominal contraction? Let me explain. The transverse abdominis is part the core and works by pulling the navel to the spine. It attaches to the right and left iliopsoas (hip flexor). When the transverse abdominis is not working well enough to support the trunk, one or both of the iliopsoas muscles may be overly recruited to do so. This compensatory over-utilization may explain why I often find painful tension in the iliopsoas in these cases. If greater iliopsoas tension develops on one side versus the other, it can lead to an asymmetrical pull on the pelvis, creating a one-sided anterior (forward) ilial rotation. This asymmetry, in turn, can create a detrimental length-tension relationship among the pelvic floor muscle fibers, which can weaken the pelvic floor's contraction.

Furthermore, I speculate that when the transverse abdominis muscle is weak, the torso may excessively call upon the pelvic floor for overall core control. The pelvic floor may compensate for the incompetent transverse abdominis muscle and become over-fatigued. The pelvic floor muscles would then work overtime to pick up the deep abdominal muscles' slack. Add an asymmetrical pelvis due to unduly recruitment of a hip flexor and overuse compounds with a mechanical disadvantage, setting the pelvic floor up for failure.

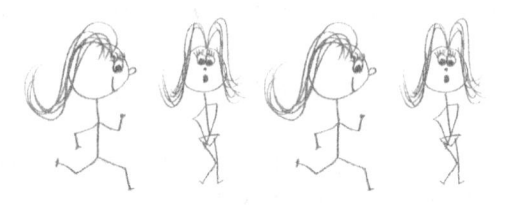

Stress Urinary Incontinence that Occurs Only with Exercise?

It's More Common Than One May Think

I have worked with a number of women who experienced stress urinary incontinence *only with exercise*. These cases had a common denominator: Difficult childbirths. The difficult childbirths either involved being in labor for up to 32 hours with extensive pushing efforts, experiencing extensive and traumatic tearing of the vaginal walls, or a combination of both.

A case in point is Jamie, a 28 year-old mother who could walk, lift, carry, transfer position, and climb and descend hills and stairs without issue, but experienced incontinence when running and when jumping with aerobics. The jolt of running and jumping rendered extensive impact on the pelvic floor. But, so did repeatedly lifting a 16-pound child. Why the incontinence with an exercise regime? New moms can resume exercising after healing from childbirth. The exercises are notably added to an already rigorous lifestyle caring for a growing baby, and all the necessary activities associated with being a mother of a young one. Perhaps the exercise *in addition* to all of the other activities performed is the proverbial straw. To ask a new mother of 5 months to stop playing the role of a mother and just exercise is out of the question. Asking her to run in the morning while the pelvic floor muscles are still fresh, versus later in the day after the pelvic floor has already been tasked, is a much more realistic option. Accumulation of physical stress with ongoing daily tasks and inadequate sleep due to a rigorous feeding cycle are confounding factors that may still disallow the pelvic floor to fully and adequately recover from a day's work. But, after *some* rest, the morning hours *may* afford a new mom exercise without incontinence until enough strength and endurance are built to avoid incontinence with all activities throughout her hectic day. Further along in the day, she may note incontinence with lifting if the pelvic floor muscles are fatigued. However, we are keeping in mind at the outset of rehabilitation what activities with the urinary control are most important to the patient. If lifting her child later in the day requires the wearing of an undergarment, but exercising earlier in the day does not, she may be very pleased, and progress will provide for the eventual urinary control with all activity despite the time of day. Helping a patient fully regain continence is the chief goal, but helping her "stay in the game" along the way to recovery is a close second.

*"You gave me my life back!
Running is my release.
Without it I was not whole.
Now, I am truly back in action!"*

On her second visit for treatment, Jamie reported significantly reduced leakage with a walk-run interval workout over the course of 30 minutes. She attributed her success to a conscious effort in Kegeling with the running, and the actual ability to Kegel strongly with the run earlier versus later in the day. She did have small episodes of incontinence, but they consisted of small drops instead of a full pad's worth of urine. Even later in the day, Jamie was able to contract around isolated episodes of intra-abdominal pressure, as with the lifting of her child, a box, or a bag of heavy items. Jamie was already "programmed" to Kegel in response to lifting's increase in intra-abdominal pressure, perhaps because her body had enough time to prepare for the continent feat. Running incontinence-free demanded a quicker reaction time of the pelvic floor. Reacting quickly to unexpected increases in abdominal pressure inherent in fast changes of position and holding repeatedly against quick jolts to the pelvic cavity required greater agility and endurance. Jamie's agility and endurance waned with fatigue. Kegeling in intervals provided the rest time Jamie's pelvic floor needed until it built endurance. Jamie practiced well-timed, isolated Kegels while hopping on two feet, then on one foot at a time, then while essentially playing hopscotch. She gradually increased the length of her hopscotch course as her pelvic floor muscle endurance allowed. Jamie's pelvic floor was on the road to gaining the agility and endurance it needed to keep her continent while out on a run!

After 6 weeks of therapy, Jamie ran to her last appointment, pushing her baby in a stroller over rolling hills without a drop of incontinence. She hugged me. And, with a tear in her eye, she emphatically stated, "You gave me my life back! Running is my release. Without it I was not whole. Now, I am truly back in action!" (P.S. I cried, too.)

While on the topic of running...running not only quickly changes one's position and provides a jolt to the abdomen and pelvic floor, it also renders the opening of one's lower extremities. Once again, the length-tension curve can come into play and the pelvic floor muscle fibers may be disadvantageously lengthened at a time when they need to perform at their best. Hence, another reason why incontinence may only occur with running or other exercises that jolt the body and open the stance of the lower extremities.

Could Estrogen Play a Role in Stress Urinary Incontinence with Exercise?

There is speculation that hormonal changes during exercise may associate with stress urinary incontinence, but as of this publication I had not found explicit research supporting such. The question I pose is this: How do we know whether it is the added intra-abdominal force or the hormonal change that invokes incontinence? For my patients who fall into this category, swimming triggers incontinence just as running and jumping do. Whether or not being immersed in water triggers the detrusor muscle to contract or the pelvic floor muscles to relax is up for debate. Nonetheless, I have had a number of patients who can perform all other activities, including those that increase intra-abdominal stress, except exercise. In a later section (entitled *Cortisol: Stress's Link to Incontinence with Exercise?*) I will discuss possible effects of cortisol on incontinence. I suspect cortisol is linked to urinary urgency at the *beginning* of a session of exercise. *Throughout* the session of exercise, however, I speculate that surges of estradiol or estrogen have an impact on stress urinary incontinence. And, this is why...

An elevated level of estradiol has been shown to correlate with a higher incidence of incontinence in women. One study supports this correlation in women between the ages of 50 and 59, which may explain incontinence in women on hormone therapy.[19] There is also an increase in estrogen premenstually and mid-cycle with ovulation.[20] Literature supports a hormonal sensitivity in the urethra's tissue.[19] Could an elevated hormonal level increase the incidence of incontinence? Quite possibly, as I have seen hormonal surges influence urinary control.

In the beginning stages of therapy, when the pelvic floor's muscle strength is not up to par, many of my patients have experienced a greater incidence of incontinence the week before menstruation. Even if patients were making gains toward continence prior to the premenstrual week, they often still noted this premenstrual regression. I speculate that a premenstrual surge of estrogen may contribute to the higher rate of incontinence. Why the premenstrual surge and not the pre-ovulatory surge? The pre-ovulatory spike in estrogen rapidly reduces with ovulation.[20] The length of time the pre-ovulatory level of estrogen is elevated may not be long enough to cause a noticeable increase in incontinence. Premenstrual water retention may also interfere with continence, as it can add pressure to the pelvic region, increasing the counter contraction required of the pelvic floor. However, despite varying levels of water retention reported, greater difficulty controlling urine flow the week before menses has been a common theme.

The good news is that once the pelvic floor becomes strong, this regression is usually not repeated, at least to the same degree. With successive estrogen surges, patients have noted difficulty contracting the pelvic floor, however the level of difficulty usually diminishes as the overall strength and agility of the pelvic floor muscles improves. According to the cases I have seen, the more automatic the strong, isolated contraction, the lesser the impact of the menstrual cycles' estrogen surges on incontinence. The potential influence of the hormonal surge is seemingly overcome by a strong pelvic floor contraction.

The association I have seen among hormonal surges and incontinence makes me wonder if there are surges of estradiol or estrogen throughout exercise or if there is a rearing of another hormone such as progesterone influencing the ability to control urination. Fatigue and repeated intra-abdominal pressure can strongly influence the control, as I have depicted previously. But, sometimes incontinence erupts even with low levels of fatigue and pressure giving me a strong hunch that, for some women, there is another factor. If so, we may have more than one reason behind exercise-induced stress urinary incontinence.

◆ ◆ ◆

Stress urinary incontinence is indeed a condition whereby one is unable to hold the pelvic floor muscles to counter intra-abdominal pressure. However, as I hope to have pointed out, there are many variables that can influence each case. The dissection of each case and the analysis of each treatment session should be an ongoing process. Communication is a necessary ingredient in the rehabilitation of incontinence. Although the same diagnosis may be given and several commonalities among cases may exist, each patient is an individual with her own story. Good communication can decode the causes of stress urinary incontinence and expedite recovery. With diligence, a life with dry undies can be regained!

Urinary Urgency and Frequency

Urinary urgency and frequency are characterized by the *need* to use the restroom before the bladder is full, otherwise leaking occurs. We are normally alerted to seek a restroom when our bladders are filled to 300-400 ml. Even with this amount of urine stored in the bladder, we can normally walk calmly to the restroom to void. When the urge suddenly strikes and results in an all out sprint to the restroom, there is a problem. When urine leakage is experienced in conjunction with the sudden urge, especially without having a full bladder, there is an even bigger problem. Frequency can follow urgency's lead to the restroom, characterizing the *need* to urinate *more often* than when the bladder is full. Therefore, urinary urgency and frequency are often partners in crime.

Having a very strong urge to void is normal when the bladder is absolutely full. We ordinarily contract our pelvic floor muscles to hold the urine and combat the detrusor's contraction. (See previous Figure 5a.) With a weak pelvic floor, a sense of urgency may strike even when the bladder is not full. The weak contraction of the pelvic floor is not strong enough to send a signal to turn off the bladder's contraction. If the pelvic floor contraction is weak, the signal is weak. If the signal is weak, the bladder's detrusor muscle contracts and pushes hard on the internal sphincter, and out rushes the urine!

A problematic sense of urgency spawns a mad dash to the restroom, even for only a small amount of urine.

Generally, we void every 3-4 hours. There are variations in normal urinary frequency, of course, due to bladder size (normally 400 to 600 ml) and the amount of liquid we consume. Sometimes, we urinate more often, as when we drink lots of fluids, or less often, as when we hold urine throughout out a night's sleep. There are certain foods and drinks, which are listed in a later section entitled *'Chemical Stimulants Can Create an Angry Bladder'*, that can irritate the bladder causing the detrusor muscle to contract regardless of the amount of urine in the bladder. These bladder irritants can stimulate detrusor contraction in normal situations. Again, it is the dire need to urinate or the leaking without the fullness that indicates a problem.

Key in the Door Syndrome

Key in the door syndrome is a condition whereby urge is controlled only until the proximity of a restroom is near. A person driving home from work with a moderately full bladder may get caught in unexpected traffic, but is able to control the urge to void…until she reaches the key to her door. Even if she stopped at an extra red light, she would be able to control that urge until that key gets into the lock…hence the title of the syndrome.

Key in the door syndrome carries over into other scenarios as well, even when there is no key, and no door. Upon sensing an urge to void while shopping, a person with *key in the door syndrome* may start to walk briskly through the store to find a restroom. Initially she can control the urge, albeit with a bit of panic. Her urge may intensify upon closing in on a restroom, and hasten her pace! Even if she starts to run, she can still control the urge and keep from leaking. Upon seeing the restroom sign, however, her control is lost. Or, she may make it all the way into the bathroom, but leak or fully lose bladder control just before she sits or squats to void. This is the same principle that applies to *key in the door syndrome.* The urge is controlled for a fair amount of time, but is ultimately the victor in the bladder battle and causes a patient to prematurely void.

The question I pose in identifying *key in the door syndrome*, however, is this: Is a patient's diagnosis of *key in the door syndrome* a problem of stress incontinence or of urgency? Is the act of getting out of the car when finally home causing stress incontinence? Is the repeated jolt of the hurried steps to the bathroom too much for the pelvic floor's endurance level to counter? Or, does the brain's micturition center prematurely send signals to the bladder that it is time to void? Quite often, it is a combination of all of the above.

The combination of stress and urge incontinence is a common occurrence, and the above scenarios predispose both. Getting out of the car and running both increase intra-abdominal pressure. This pressure pushes downward on the pelvic floor, which may already be maxed out from trying to counter a contracting bladder. Approaching a restroom, driving into one's driveway, turning a key to unlock a door all signal that a toilet is near. A premature release in inhibition from the brain's micturition center allows the detrusor to contract, and may result in the sudden urgency to void. Leaking or voiding results if the pelvic floor muscles are not strong enough to close the urethra and to send the message to halt the bladder.

The best way I have found to treat this scenario is to attack it from both angles. Strengthening the pelvic floor and effectively timing the contraction can increase the ability to counter the intra-abdominal pressure's push on the bladder. A stronger pelvic floor can also send adequate messages to halt the contraction of the bladder's detrusor muscle. The stronger the contraction, the stronger the message sent through the feedback loop. It goes a little something like this:

The stronger pelvic floor contraction →
the greater the feedback.

The greater the feedback →
the stronger the detrusor's inhibition.

The stronger the detrusor's inhibition →
the weaker the detrusor's contraction.

The weaker the detrusor's contraction →
the greater the success in controlling urgency.

Thus, by strengthening the pelvic floor, its contraction can counter the stress applied to the abdominal cavity *and* signal to halt the bladder's untimely havoc.

With urgency, the *isolated* contraction of the pelvic floor is doubly important. As with stress incontinence, contracting the abdominals is counterproductive. Increased intra-abdominal pressure results in enhanced pressure on the bladder and internal sphincter, making it even more difficult for the pelvic floor to hold against the urine's flow. This greater workload can overly exert the pelvic floor, which is already in dire need of sending signals to stop the bladder's contraction. Also, a strong contraction of the pelvic floor (and only the pelvic floor) is the trigger that signals the brain's micturition center to stop the contraction of the bladder. The pelvic floor muscles, not the abdominals, gluteals or adductors, hold the reigns over the micturition center. Therefore, the pelvic floor contraction, strong in isolation, is paramount to controlling the urge.

As with a patient who experiences only stress urinary incontinence, I help a patient with urinary urgency determine the length of time she needs to find the pelvic floor muscles and how long she is able to contract those muscles in isolation. This is the contraction duration we start with for urge control (as well as for countering stress urinary incontinence). Once again, for each length of contraction, I ask the patient to only contract as intensely as she can in isolation of the abdominals, gluteals, and adductors. Even if the intensity is minimal, even if the length of time is barely a second, isolation is key. Only with isolation is building intensity and length of hold an effective shield against incontinence. Gradually, I ask the patient to progress her home program to include practicing long, isolated Kegels for up to 10 seconds and short, pulsed holds for 2 seconds or less.

On the hunt for a restroom or in attempts to avoid an uncontrollable urge when inserting a key in the door, multiple series of 10 short pelvic floor muscle contractions of 2 seconds or less can give bursts of feedback to the micturition center to inhibit the bladder's detrusor muscle contraction. Incontinence due to urgency can be avoided by holding a Kegel with moderate force, while pulsing stronger contractions for 2 seconds or less. The pelvic floor should not be fully relaxed between the more strongly pulsed contractions. Rather, the Kegel should only be released to the level of the moderate baseline hold. Adding the short contractions are seemingly more effective in feeding the micturition center requests to inhibit the detrusor than holding the moderate Kegel alone.

However, oftentimes patients do not want to let the pelvic floor muscles relax to any degree out of fear of inappropriately timed urination. Furthermore, some patients have difficulty pulsing the pelvic floor in isolation of the abdominals. With urgency in full force, adding intra-abdominal pressure would likely stage an incontinent episode. In these cases, a constant Kegel held alone without the shorter, stronger pulses would suffice to start. With training and practice, the short pulses can be added with confidence.

Longer Kegel holds of 10 seconds should be practiced in conjunction with the shorter holds to help the pelvic floor endure long bouts of urgency. I ask patients with urinary urgency to also perform the longer holds followed by quick bursts of contraction to help counter *sudden* rises in intra-abdominal pressure that can occur with sneezing and coughing. These sudden pressure surges can tax the pelvic floor especially in times of urgency when its muscles are fiercely working to fight a strongly contracting bladder. Ideally, with restoration of control over urge incontinence, all of the demands placed on the pelvic floor muscles are addressed automatically, in a timely manner. A solid resting tone develops, short contractions send urgent messages to stop the bladder's contraction, and quick, strong bursts of contraction counter sudden jolts of intra-abdominal pressures.

Like stress urinary incontinence, timing of the pelvic floor contraction is very important. Upon sensing an urge, I encourage patients to pulse short contractions as well as possible in attempts to turn the detrusor off via the feedback loop. In a hopeful scenario, once the urge subsides, the patient can then calmly walk to the toilet. Even if the patient has not yet sensed the strong urge, but is nearing home, approaching a restroom, or unlocking the front door, performing Kegel exercises can be beneficial in keeping the urgency from developing. So, rather than "wee wee wee all the way home"... Squeeze! Squeeze! Squeeze! ...Instead.

A home exercise program is recommended to assist

with learning to contract the pelvic floor and to build its agility. (See previous Figure 14.) Figure 19 depicts the specific timing of the Kegels for urge suppression.

Figure 19. An example of a home program to help independently suppress the urge to void.

Regaining Control over Urinary Urgency and Frequency

Suppressing the urge to void: Pelvic floor contractions can suppress the urge by sending messages to the brain-bladder network to stop the bladder's contraction. It is often easier to suppress the urge in a seated position versus in a standing position. It is helpful to have a chair close to the restroom in order to practice.

When you sense the urge to urinate:
- If possible, sit down. If lying down and an urge strikes, remain in the lying position.
- Perform 10 short bursts of Kegels, only as long as you need to find the muscles and only as firmly as you can in isolation.
- Stay calm and allow the urge to subside.
- If the urge has not been suppressed, repeat 10 short Kegels.
- If lying down or seated, hold the Kegel around the transfer to the standing position.
- Calmly walk to the restroom while holding a moderate Kegel and quickly pulsing stronger Kegels. This is similar to holding a rope in your hand, clenching just enough so it does not drop, and clenching harder if someone tried to pull it out of your hand! If you are unable to release to the moderate hold without leaking, simply hold your firm contraction while making your way to the restroom.
- Void once the timing is appropriate.

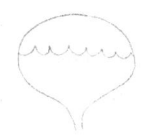

Artificially Induced Urinary Urgency... As a Treatment??

      Hearing or seeing running water can increase a sense of urinary urgency just as stepping into a warm shower can. Why? Quite possibly because these audio, visual, and tactile cues can trigger the micturition center's contraction of the bladder as if associating running water with a time to void. So, when treating, why not use running water to artificially strengthen the urge and trigger the need to exert an even stronger pelvic floor contraction to counter the urgency? Trust me, this works! By increasing the sense of urgency, we can create a strong need for the pelvic floor to not only hold back the urine stream, but also to communicate to the brain's micturition center that the bladder must stop contracting and the internal sphincter must close. Contracting the pelvic floor (Kegeling) to counter the artificially induced urgency is a challenging exercise, but it can help patients remain continent in difficult situations.

      Kate presented with a *key in the door-like* condition whereby she could control the urge only until she saw a bathroom present or knew a restroom was in close proximity. Therefore, at the start of her treatments, Kate sequentially practiced Kegeling in sitting, holding the Kegel while transferring from sit to stand, and while walking to the restroom. Once Kate was able to hold a firm baseline of a contraction, she pulsed strong holds while walking to the toilet then relaxed once voiding was timed appropriately. Once Kate mastered getting to the restroom on time in such a controlled environment, I asked Kate to hold en route to the restroom while listening to me pour water from one container to another. Listening to water flowing and seeing the restroom induced an urge that gave Kate one heck of a workout! (If I may digress, the water was then used to water the plants. I am adamant about not wasting water.) Eventually Kate was able to overcome sudden bouts of urgency with pelvic floor contractions and she became desensitized to the visual and audible urgency triggers. With further practice, Kate's sudden inappropriate urges downgraded to normally occurring, full bladder-induced urges.

    I like to simulate very difficult scenarios in the clinic so that real life seems relatively easy! Increased urgency in the presence of running water can definitely be difficult to overcome! Patients that Kegeled in the presence of running water noted a spike in difficulty in countering an urge and needed a greater pelvic floor contraction to avoid an incontinent episode. Whether the patient sees or hears the water, or is standing in a shower's flow, strong, isolated Kegels seem to break the brain's connection between water flow and untimely voiding. These advanced treatment scenarios have been very successful in affording patients urge control in some of life's most difficult situations.

1:00   2:30   4:00

Timed Voiding to Counter Urinary Urgency and Frequency

Another means of countering urge incontinence is timed voiding. Timed voiding can give the patient voluntary control over her urination frequency. The goal of timed voiding is to catch the urge before it strikes and suppress the urge before it is uncontrollable. Therefore, during the beginning stage of therapy, the patient actually urinates *more* frequently than before she started treatment. The increase in frequency is a conscious decision, though, instead of a dire need. The conscious decision to urinate gives the patient control over the voiding schedule, instead of urgency launching a surprise attack during an untimely situation. The higher urination frequency should only be at the outset of therapy. While implementing the timed voiding schedule, the patient should engage in a series of pelvic floor contractions appropriate for her condition, as previously described in the section entitled '*Key in the Door Syndrome*'. Once the urge is contained with greater pelvic floor control, the time in between the conscious voids can gradually increase. The patient's urination frequency can eventually resume normalcy and allow for voiding in accordance with a full bladder instead of a premature urge.

If a patient senses strong urgency and/or experiences leaking every hour, I recommend voluntarily going to restroom every 45 minutes. Even if the urge is not present, the patient is encouraged to go to the restroom. As long as the urge is controlled for the current interval, the patient can increase the amount of time in between voids by approximately 15 minutes. Figure 20 suggests timed voiding tips as part of a home exercise program. With a conscious decision to urinate, before the strong, uncontrollable urge strikes, voiding can occur with the release of the pelvic floor, instead of at the detrusor's will. Thus, the patient can usurp the voiding power, stripping the detrusor of its erratic and untimely contractions.

Figure 20. An example of a timed voiding regime.

Regaining Control of Urinary Urgency and Frequency

Timed voiding: Setting specific times to void throughout the day catches the urgency before it strikes.
- If you need to void once every hour, time your trip to the restroom every 45 minutes.
- After the urgency is curbed, gradually increase the voiding intervals by 15 minutes. If sudden, uncontrollable urges are still sneaking up on you, return to the more frequent voiding schedule.
- The gradual increase in time between voids can help you gain control of the voiding and eventually allow you to void in accordance with a full bladder.

✦ ◆ ✦

Tara was a patient with urgency and frequency striking every hour. This was not conducive to her work as a dental assistant whereby her presence was needed for up to 5 hours at a time for a single patient procedure. Strengthening of the pelvic floor muscles and timed voids at 45 minutes intervals gained Tara the conscious control of the void. Soon, Tara was able to hold through the 60-minute procedures. When Tara was able to hold for 75-minute periods, she continued with the gradual interval training while at home. At work, however, the voids at longer intervals sometimes coincided with a patient procedure. Therefore, I recommended that she use the restroom in between patients, even if at a higher frequency than she needed, so that the urge would not become uncontrollable during the next patient procedure. Tara soon got into the habit of voiding in between patients to curb the urges, and was still making progress at home with the gradual lengthening of voiding intervals.

Tara's urgency was soon controlled on days with procedures of up to 2 hours, but how did we address the longer stints of up to 5 hours that disallowed a restroom break? The longer holds were eventually achieved with the practice of a timed voiding schedule on her days off from work, and during working hours when her schedule allowed. In the meantime, we looked at ergonomics as means of feasibly improving her continence while tending to a patient. If possible, Tara sat down to ease the burden of gravity's push on the pelvic floor. If she needed to stand, she did so with her legs closed instead of partly opened. Standing with her legs together optimized the length-tension relationship of the pelvic floor muscle fibers. Instead of reaching and lunging, she took small steps to retrieve items, holding the objects close. Retrieving the objects in closer proximity reduced the torque applied to the abdominal cavity, thereby reducing the magnitude of intra-abdominal pressure. Lighter intra-abdominal pressure lessened the workload of the pelvic floor allowing for efficient use of energy for longer contractions of a moderate hold and stronger quick contractions for urge control. Tara did wear a pad to retain the leaking urine in case of emergencies with the longer patient procedures…but not for long. Dissecting Tara's workday allowed us to improve the efficiency of her pelvic floor's energy. With conscious voiding control, greater strength, and improved timing and agility, Tara was soon able to hold even through 4-5 hour bouts of work procedures, no sweat…or *urine*!

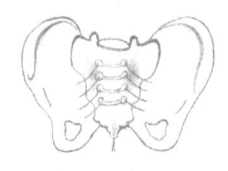

When Well-Timed, Isolated Kegels and Timed Voids Are Not Enough, Electrical Stimulation to the Rescue!

For the patients who are unable to successfully curb the urge with pelvic floor contractions, I introduce electrical vaginal stimulation. To increase the actual strength of the Kegel, I use a frequency of 50 Hz while the patient repeatedly contracts for 10 seconds and rests for 10, as I do for stress urinary incontinence. A lower frequency of 12.5 Hz is separately administered during the treatment, as this frequency can be effective in stopping the detrusor's contraction.[21] I administer the 12.5 Hz electrical vaginal stimulation while the patient performs short pelvic floor contractions. These Kegels are, of course, only as forceful as the patient can contract in isolation. Performing short Kegels while receiving the detrusor-inhibiting 12.5 Hz of stimulation may enhance the signal to the micturition center to inhibit the detrusor's overactivity, helping the patient fight the urge until the pelvic floor can do so independently.

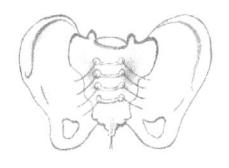

Urinary Urgency Treatment Alternatives

If the above treatment methods do not suffice, there is an alternative. I do not perform the following treatment, but I feel it is important to shed light on an alternative procedure performed by fellow medical practitioners should my methods not suffice. Treatment of urgency with an overactive detrusor muscle has reportedly been accomplished with percutateous tibial nerve stimulation and with S3 segmental nerve stimulation at low frequencies of 10-15 Hz.[22,23] Percutaneous tibial nerve stimulation involves inserting a needle electrode into the calf to send signals to the sacral nerve complex, which is responsible for detrusor stimulation. S3 stimulation involves direct sacral nerve stimulation with a needle electrode. The nerve stimulation occurs under general or local anesthesia. The electrodes modulate the nerves to control detrusor contraction. The intended result is an inhibitory effect on the detrusor to counter the urge.[22,23]

Given the successful urge control with electrically stimulated neuromodulation, what are the possibilities of success with acupuncture targeting the sacral, tibial and common peroneal nerves? I welcome the insight and research.

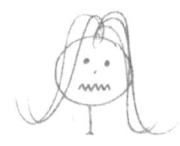

Mental Stress as a Culprit of Urinary Urgency and Frequency

I have come across several cases whereby mental stress or anxiety has lead to urinary urgency and frequency. This has also been reported in literature.[24] The stress triggering incontinence in my patients has stemmed from a myriad life's situations including new jobs, new additions to the family, pre-race jitters, and changes in a daily schedule. Furthermore, the stress associated with the inability to find a restroom or the inability to wait until an appropriate voiding time has contributed to a sense of urgency according to several of my patients. Regardless of where this mental stress originates, it can fester into incontinence.

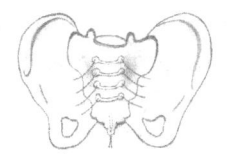

To get a bit technical...

There seems to be a paradox in the explanation for stress being a culprit of urinary urgency and frequency. In a normal situation, parasympathetic nerves stemming from levels S2-S4 increase detrusor activity and decrease internal sphincter contraction allowing for urination. Activation of sympathetic nerves stemming from T11-L2 increases the internal sphincter hold and decreases detrusor activity allowing for retention of urine.[25,26,27,28] Stress triggers the sympathetic portion of the autonomic nervous system,[29] but is associated with increases urgency and frequency. How can this be?

Speculators in the field of psychology describe stress and anxiety as small-scale 'fight-or-flight' responses. The 'fight-or-flight' response is the component that may induce urinary urgency and frequency. It has been suggested that when in 'fight-or-flight' mode, the body conserves energy to prepare for survival by shutting down parts of the brain and nervous system that are not essential to saving one's life. Holding urine does not make the survival mode cut. The micturition center of the brain, then, shuts down and causes emptying of bladder contents. The parasympathetic system may fail to bring this situation to normalcy due to overload. Experiencing an increase in anxiety, like being thrown into 'fight-or flight' mode, can disrupt the ability to hold urine if the internal sphincter muscles fail to hold.[25,26,27,28] I have noticed that a slight boost in my patients' anxiety appears to start the voiding process, making urination difficult to control, hence the heightened urgency and frequency. If the pelvic floor muscles are not strong enough to fight the urine flow and signal to stop the detrusor's contraction, urination can ensue.

For some of my patients, a sudden onset of urinary urgency may be explained by the stress and anxiety associated with changes to a daily schedule. Cassie noted particular difficulty controlling her urge when she started canoe paddling. She would void before practice, leave home, practice paddling canoe, then urgently return home, approximately 2 hours later, to void. The paddle practice was a change in her schedule as it was a new morning activity. During her treatment, Cassie visualized her new morning routine whilst Kegeling and receiving 12.5 Hz electrical vaginal stimulation. Without the stimulation, we simulated paddling, driving home, and calmly walking to the restroom, Kegeling throughout for urge control. The true test came in the clinic one day with the appearance of a common Hawai'ian 'visitor'. In Hawai'I, there are a plethora of geckos that make their homes wherever they so choose. Cassie had a profound fear of these little fellas. As she made her way to my restroom, she was halted by the presence of Mr. Gecko who snuck in under the door to my clinic and decided to scope out my restroom. With her fear of geckos inhibiting her entering the restroom, she forced herself to Kegel greater than she thought she was able. She Kegeled and successfully controlled her urgency all the way home! During the next few clinic sessions we incorporated our serendipitous scenario (with a photo of a gecko for added effect). By the next week, Cassie had role played enough to successfully counter her urgency and use the restroom in a calm and timely manner, despite any changes to her schedule.

Cortisol: Mental Stress's Link to Incontinence with Exercise?

Yet another factor in the realm of stress and anxiety is the production of cortisol, the "stress hormone".[30] Systemic cortisol levels heighten when anxiety or fear triggers its release from the adrenal glands. Physical activity, such as fleeing a frightening situation or exercising, or meditating to alleviate anxiety, can reduce the level of cortisol.[30] Without such activities to consume the cortisol, the systemic levels can remain high. It is possible that cortisol, which is linked to stress and anxiety, may be the culprit affecting detrusor activity and contributing to urinary urgency. Testing the direct effect of cortisol on the detrusor activity may shed light on the how mental stress and urinary urgency are connected.

Exercise and body temperature can have wavering effects on cortisol production. Exercise can increase cortisol production at lower body temperatures. The cortisol level can then decrease when the body reaches higher temperatures as with continued exercise.[31,32] Even having just urinated, several of my patients report a strong urge at the outset of running or otherwise exercising. They relieve themselves with a void and carry-on without an urge resurfacing. Compared to the core temperature after 'warming up', the core temperature at the start of a workout is usually relatively low. With a low core temperature, the initial strides, cycles, or jumps may enhance cortisol production. This greater concentration of cortisol may stimulate detrusor activity and create a strong urge. This extreme urge to urinate can occur despite the patient having urinated just prior to the start of the workout. As the concentration of cortisol diminishes with continued exercise and rise in core temperature, [31,32] the patient can finish her workout devoid of detrusor stimulation and urgency to urinate.

Urgency at the outset of exercise may be a normal occurrence without incontinence. I personally have noticed an occasional urge develop within 8 minutes into my run despite having just voided before starting. The urge passes after approximately 12 minutes, and even when I finish a 12-miler, I still don't have to run to the restroom. In instances such as mine, perhaps a strong pelvic floor counters the urge until the body temperature rises and depletes the cortisol concentration.

My suspected correlation between cortisol and urinary urgency differs from my hypothesized estrogen/estradiol effect on stress urinary incontinence. My estrogen/estradiol hypothesis suggests that the hormonally influenced stress urinary incontinence occurs throughout a bout of exercise. I suspect that cortisol causes an urge only until its production decreases with elevated body temperature. With continued exercise, cortisol levels are likely low and thusly do not trigger the bladder's detrusor muscle to contract. Cortisol's stimulation of urgency at the outset of exercise, like estrogen and/or estradiol's effect on stress incontinence, is *only* speculation, and I welcome research in this arena.

Until such research is found, allow me to present one example of my many cases leading to my conclusion. Hillary presented with stress urinary incontinence and urinary urgency. She was able to keep continent with a single activity. However, with repeated activity, the pelvic floor became easily fatigued. Running was a chief concern. Hillary ran not only to improve her athletic self, but also to relieve her daily stress. In this case, because she was not able to run without stress urinary incontinent episodes, she opted to run in small intervals. The small intervals did not target all stress relief, but they were certainly better than not running at all. Hillary noted strong urges with the interval running with only a small amount of urine to void. This had not been the case when she could run her full 8 miles without intervals. Cortisol levels likely rose at the outset of her run, and quite possibly remained high throughout her interval workout. Her normal 8-mile run likely would have elevated her body temperature and decreased the cortisol levels, but the shorter intervals of running with rest in between may not have elevated her body temperature enough to lessen the cortisol production. The excessive amounts of cortisol may have irritated the detrusor muscle just enough to set it into contractions. Hillary did not have adequate strength and endurance of the pelvic floor to hold against the flow of urine with added intra-abdominal pressure. Furthermore, her weak pelvic floor contraction seemingly was not enough to signal the micturition center to stop the detrusor's contraction. Without enough exercise to consume the cortisol and without enough pelvic floor strength to counter cortisol's alleged stimulation of the bladder's detrusor muscle, a downward spiral into incontinence ensued. (See Figure 21.)

With rehabilitative efforts to lengthen her running intervals, Hillary resumed her full 8-mile run without stress urinary incontinence. Her urgency dwindled as well, with greater pelvic floor strength, and possibly with resuming a workout that depleted cortisol levels and its potential stimulation of the bladder's detrusor muscle.

Figure 21. An initial evaluation written for a patient with urinary urgency particularly upon commencing exercise, and with stress urinary incontinence.

Diagnoses: Urinary urgency at the commencement of exercise and stress urinary incontinence.

Upon evaluation, the following were noted:
1. Patient reports gradual onset of stress urinary incontinence ~ 2/1/04. Patient notes a particularly strong urge a few minutes after setting out to run, and reports leaking with sneezing and coughing.
2. Patient has difficulty isolating pelvic floor from gluteals. She is able to hold her pelvic floor, but only for ~ 3 seconds in standing, and ~ 5 seconds in sitting.
3. Patient is able to hold the pelvic floor contraction against the intra-abdominal pressure added when holding a 3 pound object, but only for ~2 seconds in standing.
4. Patient is unable to hold the pelvic floor while running and walking, and while repeatedly transferring from sitting to standing,
5. A key factor in her recovery is the ability to counter added intra-abdomnal pressure in standing, without the assistance of a chair to support the pelvic floor, and to hold a Kegel while sustaining a jolt of intra-abdominal pressure as with running, sneezing, and coughing.
6. Timing of the pelvic floor contraction (Kegel) has commenced and will continue to be integrated into therapy. We are working to regain the automatic nature of a true Kegel.
7. The higher cortisol level at the start of a run (due to a lower body temperature) and the anxiety stemming from the thought of possibly having an incontinent episode while running may both interfere with the ability to keep continent.
8. Interval training is advised in order to run with minimal stress urinary incontinence.
9. Pelvic floor strengthening aims to improve endurance for a full run without incontinence and to combat the urgency possibly

potentiated by cortisol.
10. Should electrical stimulation and/or electrical biofeedback be appropriate and necessary, measures will be taken.

Plans/Goals
1. Independent with home exercise program.
2. Isolation of pelvic floor contraction.
3. Independent timing of pelvic floor hold for countering all incontinent episodes.
4. No episodes of stress urinary incontinence or urgency.

Chemical Stimulants Can Create an Angry Bladder

Nutrients can have a profound effect on the bladder. Some of the foods and beverages we consume can chemically trigger the detrusor muscle to contract, creating a sense of urinary urgency. I have provided a list of foods and beverages that may cause such urgency, and a list of possible alternatives for those affected. Some foods and beverages are not considered irritants unless a large quantity of such is consumed. And, of course, the level of irritation is patient dependent. The chemical irritants have a tendency to trigger detrusor contraction, but each person can be affected to different degrees. (See Figure 22.)

Figure 22. Bladder stimulants and alternatives.[33]

A prematurely stimulated, angry bladder may result from consuming the following: [33]

Alcohol	Large Apples
Citrus Fruits And Juices	Carbonated Beverages
	Coffee
Spicy Foods, i.e. Chili Peppers	Cranberries
	Grapes
Chocolate	Strawberries
Avocado	Lentils
Tea	Fava Beans
Raw Onions	Artificial Sweeteners
Vitamins	Sour Cream
Cheese	Mayonnaise
	Vitamins With Aspartate

Alternative items for a calmer bladder include: [33]

Late Harvest Wines	Highly Roasted Coffee
Blueberries	Low Acid Tomatoes
Carob	Small Apples
White Chocolate	Almonds
Cooked Onions	Pine Nuts
Sun Tea	Peanuts

With Chemically Induced Urinary Urgency, Drink More Water:

Another Paradox?

It is important to note that my intention is not to keep patients from eating and drinking the irritants that are staples of nutrition. I do, however, recommend drinking a glass of water when consuming them. Increasing water intake can dilute the bladder irritants and may potentially ease the detrusor's chemical-induced premature contraction. Highly concentrated urea can develop from processing ingested items with a low dose of water. This concentrated urea can also serve as a strong bladder irritant, which may cause a person to have to void more frequently due to the chemical stimulation of the detrusor. Drinking more water to reduce incontinence may seem like a paradox, as it will lead to a fuller bladder. However, the ensuing urgency and frequency of urination would be due to a *full* bladder, which is completely normal, instead of a minimally filled bladder contracting uncontrollably around a mere puddle of irritants.

Chemical irritants may affect many bladders without causing incontinence. A weakened pelvic floor that is unable to counter the bladder's resulting contraction is often the link to uncontrollable urgency and frequency. Strengthening and agility training is recommended to combat the urgency and frequency. But, to improve upon overall incontinence in the short run, I recommend consuming a glass of water to dilute irritating ingredients. The added water can put out the proverbial fire, if you will. This can help to control the urge incontinence until the strength of the pelvic floor is able to do so.

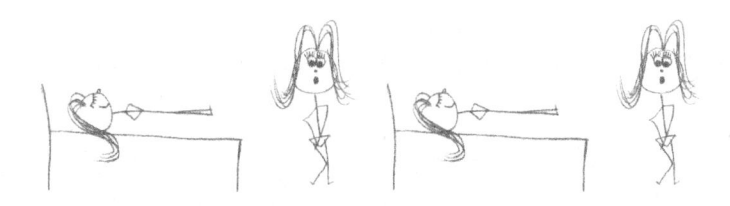

Nocturia:
Nightly Urinary Frequency

Nocturia is the nagging need to frequently use the restroom while attempting to sleep, which is usually at night, hence the name. (For the purposes of this book, I will refer to sleeping hours at night, and waking hours during the day.) The bladder's detrusor muscle does not go to sleep. And, if the pelvic floor muscles cannot counter urinary urgency with strong contractions, frequent trips to the restroom can make sound sleeping impossible.

There is a possible contributor to excessive voiding at night, which, interestingly enough, does not involve a problematic pelvic floor. The frequent trips to the restroom at night may be due to the elimination of excess fluids accumulated in the lower extremities during the daytime. With our legs in a dependent or downward position, fluid pooling may occur if the leg muscles do not actively contract enough to circulate the fluid out of the lower extremities. When lying in a horizontal position, the fluid that collected can circulate out of the lower limbs, to the lymphatic drainage system, and eventually to the bladder. With large volumes of fluid circulating out of the lower limbs, frequent restroom visits may be inevitable.

The fluid retention can be curbed with modifications to diet and with an increase in water intake. Many people are told to stop drinking water after 6 pm to avoid awakening frequently to urinate. This may very well be the *cause* of awakening. Not only may more fluid pool without being flushed, the concentration of urea in the urine may increase. Once again, a high concentration of urea can irritate the bladder, causing the detrusor muscle to contract prematurely. Therefore, contrary to popular suggestion, I recommend imbibing a steady amount of water, even into the evening. This can help to keep fluid flushing during the waking hours, and urea concentration below a level that would irritate the bladder and cause untimely detrusor contraction.

Should nocturia be an extension of diurnal frequency, timed voiding in the waking hours and Kegeling just before bed can help to curb the urgency. Kegeling before bed can put patients in the mind set to control the urge with pulsed pelvic floor contractions, strongly stimulating the feedback loop to counter the premature detrusor muscle contractions. Voluntarily awakening to time the voids during the night can also effectively help patients retake control of the bladder. Although awakening to an alarm set throughout the night to time voiding before the urgency strikes is initially more disruptive, in time it can help patients resume a normal sleeping and voiding pattern. The frequent awakening due to urgency is also disruptive, and provides no end to the frustrating nocturia. Awakening one or two extra times per night in the short run can improve control of the bladder to make way for a normal night's sleep in the long run.

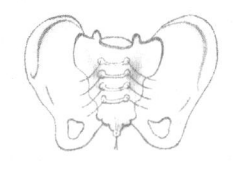

Incomplete Voiding

Urinary urgency and frequency are often found in conjunction with incomplete voiding. With incomplete voiding, a patient has difficulty fully eliminating urine from the bladder. The detrusor muscle may inadequately contract and the internal sphincter may inadequately open, or the detrusor's contraction and the internal sphincter's opening may be mistimed. Oftentimes the patient stops the urine stream prematurely or inadequately relaxes the pelvic floor when trying to void. With residual urine in the bladder, the brain may think the bladder is still in *'go mode'*. Therefore a few minutes later, the patient may need to rush into the bathroom again, oftentimes with extreme urgency, to void those last drops.

There are times when urgency strikes despite having just used the restroom that is quite normal. Upon emptying a full bladder, i.e. upon awakening in the morning, we may find ourselves quickly returning to void about 10-20 minutes later. Urine trickles from the kidneys through the ureters and into the bladder. When the bladder becomes full, and the amount of urine collected cannot fit in the bladder, the urine backlogs in the ureters until space becomes available in the bladder. In this scenario, the bladder is metaphorically a jammed freeway and the ureters are the onramps. The urine waiting to enter the bladder is the trail of cars backed up on the onramps. Just as the trail of cars can move onto the freeway once space becomes available, the urine in the ureters can trickle into the bladder once voiding makes space. However, the urine backlogged in the ureters can enter the bladder when the micturition center and bladder are still in *go mode*. Strong pelvic floor muscles can counter the bladder's detrusor contraction when a second void is not desirable, but for a person with difficulty contracting, incontinence may ensue.

Here is a scenario to help put incomplete voiding into perspective. Picture oneself all bundled up whilst camping in the woods on a cold night at 13,500 feet above sea level. Nature calls and urine is knocking on the internal sphincter's door. Without knowing for certain what creatures are lurking in the dark, one might decide to heed the call of the bladder next to a nearby bush rather than walk all the way to the outhouse. Half way through voiding, a creature appears in the distance. As the creature moves closer, one stops the voiding prematurely in order to scurry into the hut protecting oneself from the wild. Sure enough falling back to sleep is not on the agenda, as the bladder, despite being only partially full, is once again asking for alleviation. *Go mode* is still in effect and an urge resurfaces. This is a normal response to the situation at hand…Trust me!

In the above scenario, the urine stream's interruption is likely partially voluntary and partially autonomic in nature. The pelvic floor muscles close the external sphincter to halt the stream instead of allowing urine to seep on the way back to the hut. There isn't enough *fright*, which would normally result in full void with a loss of urine control, but there is likely enough *stress* to halt the bladder's detrusor muscle contraction and close the internal sphincter prematurely. Once nestled in a comfortable space, stress disappears, and takes its effect on the autonomic nervous system with it. With urine trapped in the bladder, reduced sympathetic activity allows the urge to resume.

Some cases of incomplete voiding, therefore, may stem from a level of stress higher than which the patients are generally accustomed to, but lower than that of a small-scale 'fight-or-flight' situation. Whereas the 'fight-or-flight' situation would increase voiding potential,[25,26,27,28] the stress level in these cases may increase the autonomic nervous system's sympathetic activity.[29] Drawing from the previous discussion on autonomic involvement in urinary control, in the section entitled *'Mental Stress as a Culprit of Urinary Urgency and Frequency'*, low doses of sympathetic activity can weaken the contraction of the bladder's detrusor muscle and close the internal sphincter.[25,26,27,28] In a situation whereby low levels of stress associate with incomplete voiding, a patient may begin to urinate, but stop prematurely due to sympathetic overactivity and parasympathetic underactivity.[29] With residual urine in the bladder, *go mode* may still be in effect. Urgency may arise moments later, and leaking may occur if the pelvic floor muscles cannot control the urine stream and a restroom is out of reach.

Engaging in activities that add pressure to the bladder while in *go mode* strengthens the urge to void. After the insufficient void, leaking may occur as soon as the patient stands up from sitting on the toilet, due to the increased abdominal pressure with the transferring of position. Leaking after the insufficient void is especially probable with activities such as running, lifting or carrying heavy objects, climbing over walls, etc. The added intra-abdominal pressure associated with these activities presses on the bladder, which is already overtaxing the pelvic floor, and plays the role of the proverbial straw.

With an incomplete void, often patients speak of dribbling or of a weak stream. The stream may even commence normally, but then trickle for minutes, instead of for a few seconds. An untimely contraction of the pelvic floor muscles may pinch or partially pinch the stream. This mistimed contraction can inhibit the detrusor's complete contraction through the inhibitory feedback loop. Furthermore, an excessively strong resting tone in the pelvic floor can send a constant message to the brain to at least partially inhibit the detrusor's contraction. The detrusor's contraction, in this scenario, may not be as strong as it needs to be to produce a normal urine stream. The combination of the partially inhibited detrusor contraction and the incomplete relaxation of the pelvic floor muscles can birth a weak, intermittent, urine stream and a bladder left partially unemptied.

To put difficulty voiding into perspective, try urinating while in a partially squatted position instead of relaxing in a seated position. In a partial squat, sometimes it is difficult to release the Kegel muscles to start the urine flow. Once released, the flow is often slow and weak likely due to an incomplete release of the pelvic floor muscles. A potential explanation for the inadequate pelvic floor muscle release is its engagement as a core stabilizer while in the partially squatted position. It may take extra effort to actively release the pelvic floor muscles to empty the bladder when the stability of the trunk calls upon the pelvic floor for core control. For patients with difficulty voiding, the pelvic floor muscles often do not fully release even when the core is not in high demand, as when seated comfortably on a toilet.

Deployment in a war zone can set the stage for incomplete voids, potentially leading to urinary urgency and frequency. I had the opportunity to work with a patient named Dana upon her return from deployment in Afghanistan. Changes in schedule, elevated levels of daily stress, and abrupt, low scale 'fight-or-flight' experiences all likely contributed to Dana's case of incontinence. By gaining control of an isolated Kegel, learning to fully relax the pelvic floor at appropriate times, and timing her voiding schedule to minimize urgency, Dana reclaimed control of her bladder. Post-traumatic stress disorder is widely prevalent in this day and age. Urinary incontinence may very well stem from such. Although the patient may have physically left the stressful environment, the environment can live within the patient. It is helpful to explain that it may take longer to rehabilitate the post-traumatic stress-induced incontinence, but with a strong patient-clinician team, continence can be had.

Relaxing the pelvic floor is not an easy task for some, but thinking about a contraction in reverse helps. A reverse Kegel is a concentrated relaxation of the pelvic floor muscles. There is an opening sensation that gives way to relaxation. The reverse Kegel may be enhanced by lightly blowing[29b] through pursed lips as if blowing through a flute. The light exhalation is calming and relaxing, promoting relaxation and release of the pelvic floor. The blowing also places a light amount of intra-abdominal pressure on the bladder. The added intra-abdominal pressure enhances the detrusor's stretch reflex to contract more strongly against the internal sphincter, pushes the urine out of the bladder through the urethra, and eases the opening of the external sphincter. Even when not in a restroom attempting to void, patients often find it is easier to relax the pelvic floor with light exhalation. Let's try it. As long as you do not have to urinate, think about opening the pelvis's orifices, and relax the pelvic floor muscles as you slowly but firmly exhale. You will most likely find that relaxing the muscles occurs in the opposite sequence of contracting. The anterior muscles around the urethra and vagina relax first, and the posterior muscles around the anus relax second. Oftentimes it takes multiple steps to fully relax, but eventually these steps blend into one smooth release.

It may take quite a bit of concentration for patients to relax the pelvic floor. A helpful technique is to contract the pelvic floor in isolation before relaxing to reinforce the region being targeted. After contracting, there is a lag time between the voluntary contraction and resumption of guarding. Clinicians, this lag time is the time to cue the patient to gently exhale to relax. The patient then learns this timing to perform the contract-relax sequence independently.

The relaxation may seem complete until the patient is asked to relax again. The patient may realize she has not fully released after the first release, and the second. Fully releasing may take several attempts. I often ask the patient to follow these 4 steps:

1. Contract the pelvic floor muscles.
2. Gently exhale[29b] and concentrate on releasing the pelvic floor.
3. Exhale[29b] a second time to release.
4. Exhale[29b] a third time to release.

Following the 4 steps to release the pelvic floor muscles can be very effective while sitting on a large therapy ball. The contour of the ball fits nicely beneath the pelvic floor, allowing the patient to sense the pressure of the ball against the perineum and the undersurface of the pelvis. Changes in this pressure act as a tactile cue that relaxation is occurring. The pressure on the perineum and pelvis slowly moves downward and outward with concentrated relaxation. This exercise is easier to 'feel' than to verbally describe. If you have access to a therapy ball, sit on it and release the pelvic floor muscles. You will likely sense the pressure changes as your muscles relax. Given the conical shape the ball assumes while the patient is sitting on it and the slow downward and outward flow of tactile sensation, I have named this reverse Kegel exercise the *lava flow*.

There are a number of other helpful strategies to promote fully voiding. Figure 23 is a list that I share with patients.

Figure 23. Helpful hints to help relax the pelvic floor muscles and fully void.

Relaxing the Pelvic Floor To Release Tension and To Fully Void

1. Blow[29b] when you go. When voiding, blow air through your mouth as if you are blowing gently into a flute, through semi-pursed lips.

2. After voiding, stand up then sit down or walk around the bathroom, then try voiding again. Again, blow[29b] when you go. Standing from a seated position and walking will apply intra-abdominal pressure to the bladder as will the blowing previously described. Standing and walking put greater forces on the bladder should such additional forces be needed.

3. Listen to running water, or think *water falls!*

4. Step into a warm shower or bath, then try voiding. Again, blow[29b] when you go!

Why do the aqueous visual, audio, and tactile cues complement a full void? Like triggering an urge in cases of urinary urgency, my answer is that hearing running water or visualizing rushing rapids may trigger the micturition center to stimulate the detrusor's contraction. The contraction will lead to urination as long as the pelvic floor muscles cooperate.

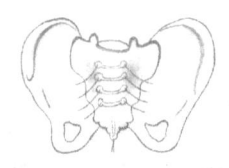

Electrical Stimulation Revisited, at a Higher Frequency

Electrical vaginal stimulation at a 200 Hz frequency can assist in relaxing the pelvic floor in women presenting with incomplete void.[12] The 200 Hz stimulation utilized in conjunction with the previously described release techniques can help to optimize the release of the pelvic floor muscles if the relaxation methods do not work alone. While undergoing stimulation, the patient should concentrate on relaxing the pelvic floor, utilizing the sequential breathing techniques, and/or thinking *"water falls"* to associate running water with the ability to openly void. The combination of techniques can help promote voiding with a strong stream versus a weak, intermittent flow stopped prematurely by jittery or tense muscles that have difficulty releasing their contraction.

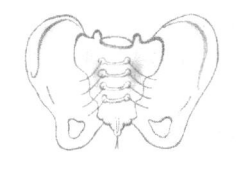

Mixed Incontinence and the Association of Incomplete Voids

Now things start to get complicated.
It is time to dig for answers outside the box ...

Mixed incontinence is a term used to describe cases whereby patients encounter stress urinary incontinence as well as urinary urgency and frequency. Mixed incontinence is quite common among patients having difficulty contracting the pelvic floor muscles and timing those contractions appropriately. Weakened or fatigued pelvic floor muscles ineffectively counter intra-abdominal pressures with stress urinary incontinence, and fail to signal the inhibition of the bladder's detrusor with urinary urgency and frequency. Poor pelvic floor muscle control can therefore lead to wet nuisances and uncontrollable urges on a frustratingly frequent basis.

As with stress urinary incontinence, catching mixed incontinence early is advantageous. Lily presented with stress urinary incontinence in the early stages, noting incontinence with sneezing and coughing, and an inability to hold while sitting from standing. She did not leak when walking on level surfaces, but she did struggle to hold continent when stepping up and down stairs. Lily reportedly needed to make the mad dash to the restroom within 5 minutes of sensing an urge, and within 5-10 minutes of having just used the restroom. The void was not usually that of a full bladder of 300-600 ml. Interestingly, Lily also initially had difficulty fully releasing the pelvic floor muscles, disallowing a full void. Her pelvic floor muscles appeared to be guarded. Incorporating a simple *blow when you go* technique as when blowing through pursed lips, Lily was able to fully void. Furthermore, after 2 days of actually fully voiding, she was able to hold the pelvic floor contraction in isolation for 10 seconds or greater, through sneezes and transfers, and while stepping up and down a step. Lily's mixed incontinence was caught while she still had some control of her pelvic floor muscles and the ability to avoid some leaking. Tackling her condition early expedited her learning of the isolated pelvic floor contraction, its appropriate timing, and its necessary release.

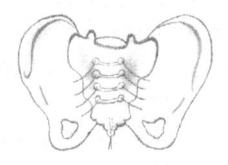

Pelvic Floor Relaxation as Rehabilitation's Driving Force

Appropriately timed, isolated Kegels were necessary for Lily to conquer mixed incontinence, however the relaxation of the pelvic floor muscles was the dominant force. Once Lily fully relaxed the pelvic floor, she completely voided with success. With a full void, her body cycled out of *go mode* and urgency and frequency ceased. In addition, the pelvic floor muscles relaxed and moved into a recovery phase. Such recovery time gave the pelvic floor muscles time to recharge as they were likely over-fatigued. This recovery time was instrumental in readying the pelvic floor to react when called upon not only to stop an urge, but to also counter the intra-abdominal force of a sneeze with a strong, tetanic contraction. Full relaxation cycled Lily out of her state of over-exertion and fully released the bladder contents. Ultimately it was the *relaxation training* that resolved urinary urgency, reduced frequency, and gave adequate rest to the pelvic floor muscles, which enabled Lily to counter the forces associated with stress urinary incontinence. (See Figure 24.)

Figure 24. An initial evaluation of a patient with mixed incontinence and incomplete void.

Diagnoses: Mixed urinary incontinence compounded by incomplete void.

Upon evaluation, the following were noted:
1. Patient reports insidious onset of urinary urgency ~ 10/26/13. Patient reports urgency, difficulty holding urine, as well as difficulty fully voiding. Incomplete void likely contributes to urgency and frequency.
2. As expected with an incomplete void, patient presents with difficulty relaxing the pelvic floor muscles. She also has difficulty contracting the pelvic floor in isolation of the abdominals after ~ 3 seconds.
3. With difficulty relaxing, the pelvic floor muscles may be in a state of fatigue. Attempting to further contract against an urge, a laugh, or a sneeze is unsuccessful.
4. Patient reports urinating at least once per hour.
5. Patient reports having a strong urgency without having a full bladder and having strong urges 5-10 minutes after having used the restroom. Urinary retention appears to contribute to the frequency.
6. Techniques to fully void and cues to contract and relax the pelvic floor muscles especially in isolation from the abdominals have commenced and will continue.
7. Should electrical stimulation and/or electrical biofeedback be appropriate and necessary, measures will be taken.

Plan/Goals
1. Independent with home exercise program.
2. Pelvic floor muscle contraction isolated.

3. Independent timing of pelvic floor contraction for countering stress urinary incontinence.
4. Independent timing of pelvic floor contraction for curbing urgency.
5. Complete void and relaxation of pelvic floor.
6. No episodes of incontinence.

◆

I will now address the importance of fully relaxing the pelvic floor in greater detail. Similar to Lily, Anna appeared to have a weakened pelvic floor, presenting with stress urinary incontinence and urinary frequency. Anna reported leaking urine with multiple sneezes and when lifting multiple bags groceries. She also reported a need to urinate every hour, despite not having a full bladder. Anna was able to contract against a light to moderate flow of urine, but not against a strong stream. Her difficulty countering the strong stream and the repetitive additions of intra-abdominal pressure was *not* due to weakness, however. On the contrary, Anna *was* strong enough to do so, but her muscles were at a constant state of fatigue. Anna's muscle fatigue mimicked sheer weakness. Why the fatigue? Because Anna was not able to fully relax the pelvic floor. Excessive use at a moderate to high level of contraction caused fatigue in her pelvic floor muscles. The resultant state of fatigue disallowed her to muster the strength to hold against multiple sneezes and coughs, and against repetitive lifting. Learning to relax the pelvic floor was crucial to the muscles' rest and recovery from exertion. Once Anna learned to fully relax the pelvic floor and gain voluntary control of the contraction, she was able to contract against activities that repeatedly added intra-abdominal pressure.

To shed light on Anna's situation, here is a scenario that will put her pelvic floor fatigue into perspective. A similar case of muscle fatigue would occur if a person held her elbow at 90 degrees with a pineapple in her hand all day. After 12 hours, if a watermelon were dropped on top of the pineapple, the person's arm would likely straighten, and down would fall the pineapple and the watermelon. The arm's biceps muscles, in such a fatigued state, would likely fail when the extra load was applied. If the watermelon was dropped and the person had not been holding the pineapple all day, chances are she would be able to hold it. Anna's constant, moderately high contraction (like carrying the pineapple) fatigued her pelvic floor muscles causing failure to hold when added stress (like the watermelon) demanded a stronger contraction. Failure of the pelvic floor (like the biceps) was fatigue-induced, not due to outright weakness.

Anna's difficulty relaxing the pelvic floor also, not surprisingly, disallowed a full void. The constant state of tension made it difficult to relax the muscles, as the fibers had likely shortened. (Think back to holding a pineapple all day. Those biceps would be tense and taut making the full extension (straightening) of the elbow painful and difficult.) Once Anna was able to relax and voluntarily contract her muscles, she gained adequate control over her urination. She achieved a normalized resting tone in her pelvic floor for urinary control with low level activity and was able to produce stronger contractions when countering a sneeze or cough (the metaphorical watermelons). Her muscles were also conditioned to relax adequately to fully void. Full relaxation, therefore, was integral in resolving Anna's urinary frequency and stress incontinence.

A similar and equally interesting case arose when a patient attempted to fend off stress urinary incontinence with her version of a Kegel, but instead created a state of urinary confusion! With the onset of mild stress urinary incontinence, Beatrice took it upon herself to attempt Kegel contractions. She was able to contract the pelvic floor, but only in conjunction with the abdominals. Contracting the abdominals created intra-abdominal pressure. This pressure compressed the bladder, giving it a sense of fullness. This sense of fullness, albeit false, then triggered the bladder's detrusor muscle to contract. The pelvic floor contraction pulsated messages to the micturition center to stop bladder contractions and consequently stop urine flow. But the co-contraction of the abdominals created a sense of fullness, which once again caused the detrusor to contract to void. Thus, a confused state of *stop and go, stop and go* replaced a smoothly streaming urine flow.

When Beatrice realized her own version of a Kegel was not curbing her incontinence, she sought my assistance. I taught her to isolate the pelvic floor by asking her to simulate stopping the urine stream while sitting on a cushioned chair and placing her hand on her abdominals. This way she could feel her pelvic floor muscles *lift* off the chair and feel her abdominals tighten when they were wrongfully co-contracting. With a few attempts, Beatrice could hold a true Kegel in isolation of the abdominals, but only for shorts bouts of 2-3 seconds, and only with a light force. Longer holds and greater force induced the abdominal co-contraction. To overcome the co-contraction, I helped Beatrice gradually strengthen the isolated Kegel with slow increases in force, and gradual increases in duration. Electrical vaginal stimulation set at 50 Hz cued the pelvic floor's whereabouts and enhanced its contraction, allowing Beatrice to more strongly Kegel in isolation. Beatrice's home exercises included the *tampon trick*, which complemented her clinic treatments by cuing where to contract in order to Kegel correctly. Within 2 weeks of therapy, Beatrice learned to strongly contract the pelvic floor muscles in isolation, repeatedly, for 10 seconds or more.

Beatrice's own attempts to Kegel before seeking therapy seemed to overly exert the pelvic floor. The abdominals' co-contraction forcefully applied intra-abdominal pressure, which likely strained the pelvic floor muscles attempting to counter it. This strain correlated with the pelvic floor muscles' guarded state and Beatrice's inability to completely void. The *stop and go* scenario described above likely emerged from an inability to completely relax a strained pelvic floor.

To help her overcome the pelvic floor muscle guarding, I taught Beatrice the *lava flow* exercise and the 4-step release, and administered 200 Hz electrical vaginal stimulation. By performing the exhalation exercises while receiving the 200 Hz stimulation and as home exercises, Beatrice's pelvic floor muscles learned to relax to allow for full voids and muscle recovery. After a couple of weeks, Beatrice's newly acquired pelvic floor control translated into solid, proactive Kegeling. By truly Kegeling and fully releasing, Beatrice could resume her efforts to minimize stress incontinence without overstraining and without compromising a full stream to void in completion.

Mandy was a combination of Anna's case (overly fatigued pelvic floor, stress urinary incontinence and urinary frequency) and Molly's case (pelvic asymmetries and stress urinary incontinence). Mandy presented with pelvic floor muscle fatigue *and* weakness. Muscle fatigue stemmed from a constantly over-exerted, guarded pelvic floor. Pelvic floor weakness associated with the disadvantageous length-tension relationship derived from pelvic asymmetries. Adding complexity to her case,

Mandy retained fluid in her lower extremities by day. When lying down to sleep, the fluid draining from her legs repeatedly filled her bladder, and Mandy awakened to frequently void throughout the night. Altogether, Mandy's pelvic floor muscle guarding and pelvic asymmetries gave rise to incomplete void, urinary frequency and urgency, and stress urinary incontinence. Inadequate diurnal lymphatic drainage carried her urinary frequency into the night. Mandy was already battling mixed incontinence with a weak, fatigued pelvic floor. Not sleeping soundly due to frequent nighttime trips to the restroom added exhaustion to the 'mix'. (See Figure 25.)

Figure 25. An example of an evaluation of a complicated patient with incomplete void, mixed incontinence, pelvic malalignment, and fluid retention.

Diagnoses: Mixed incontinence, incomplete void, nocturia complicated by ilia rotation and elevation and lymphatic blockage.

Upon evaluation, the following were noted:
1. Patient reports a gradual onset of mixed incontinence ~ 9/1/08, with progressive worsening.
2. Patient reports urinary leakage with most activities and especially with sneezing, coughing, changing position, and walking. Patient reports urgency to void without having a full bladder, and often senses the urgency within 5 minutes of having just voided. Patient urinates frequently during the day, averaging 2 voids per 60-90 minutes. Patient also awakens every 1-2 hours to void at night.
3. Patient reports pain in the lumbar and pelvic regions.
4. Pelvic pain was noted in conjunction with hip flexor tension greater on the right versus the left. This correlated with right anterior ilial rotation.
5. Tension in the right greater than left lumbar paraspinals correlates with right ilial elevation.
6. The patient also presents with lumbar degenerative disc disease, which further predisposes ilial elevation.

7. Rotation and elevation likely contribute to difficulty contracting the pelvic floor with their inherent effect of a disadvantageous length-tension relationship among the pelvic floor muscle fibers.
8. Furthermore, tension is noted in the pelvic floor muscles. Such guarding correlates with urinary retention and incomplete void. Incomplete voids correlate with urgency and frequency.
9. Patient reports swelling in bilateral lower extremities. Tension in the gracilis and hip flexors is significant and correlates with likely compression of lymph nodes and ducts in the lower extremities. Such compression likely compromises fluid mobility, leading to swelling.
10. Nocturia will be addressed with urge control techniques as well as attention to inadequate lymphatic drainage.
11. Manual therapy will complement lumbar-pelvic stabilization in reconciling pelvic asymmetries.
12. Stabilization is recommended with eventual full core control. Because abdominal contraction increases incontinence, we will commence only with the core's pelvic floor portion until incontinence improves.
13. Electrical stimulation and/or electrical biofeedback will be implemented as appropriate.

Plan/Goals
1. Independent with home exercise program.
2. Fluid retention addressed with gracilis and hip flexor muscle tension release.
3. Strengthening of an isolated pelvic floor contraction to counter stress urinary incontinence.
4. Ilial symmetry stabilized.
5. Full voids.
6. Voiding without unnecessary urgency every 3-4 hours, or in accordance with fluid intake.

◆

When cases are complicated like Mandy's, I find it best to analyze how the individual components of the case interact, then address each portion as a single case. I recommend carefully tending to each single diagnosis in manners that do not hinder the improvement of the other components. The stabilization of the pelvic floor is a perfect example of how we should circumspectly consider the interactions of each component. As stated in previous sections (including *'Asymmetries Often Underlie a Mechanical Disadvantage of the Pelvic Floor'*, *'Treating Pelvic Asymmetries'*, and *'Patients with Stress Urinary Incontinence Trudged into My Care, but with Rehabilitation, They Danced Out'*) the core's co-contraction of the deep abdominals with the pelvic floor that is needed to hold lumbar-pelvic (low back and pelvic) symmetry can interfere with the isolation of the pelvic floor needed to maintain continence. Once the pelvic floor isolation is established, the patient may be taught to contract the transverse abdominis *with* the pelvic floor. The isolated contraction of the pelvic floor also assists its own relaxation. With the proper cuing, relaxation is maximized just after the contraction, before the guarding has a chance to resurge. Understanding each piece and its role in the diagnostic weave is crucial to ensure all the pieces are fixed. The newly repaired pieces can then successfully blend to create a healthier, rehabilitated patient.

Mandy overcame all maladies with treatments that addressed each piece of her overall condition. Treatments were implemented after deciphering how each piece interfered with the others. Manual therapy to the low back and hip flexors, and stretches to promote alignment addressed the ilial asymmetries. (See previous Figure 16b.) Fluid retention was addressed with manual therapy to the hip flexors and the gracilis (the inner thigh muscle) in order to release the compressive force these muscles placed on the lymphatic system. Electrical vaginal stimulation at a frequency of 50 Hz complemented Mandy's Kegeling, helping her overcome stress urinary incontinence. At a frequency of 12.5 Hz, the stimulation assisted in resolving urinary urgency. At 200 Hz, the stimulation helped reduce the pelvic floor's muscle guarding to allow for a complete void. The isolated pelvic floor contraction addressed the incontinence. After Mandy mastered the isolated Kegel, integration of the full core held the ilia in alignment. Taking each piece of the puzzle apart and addressing it, then putting all the rehabilitated pieces together resolved Mandy's incontinence on all occasions. This dissection also rehabilitated the underlying contributors, which were problems needing attention regardless of whether they had contributed to incontinence...We fed a whole lot of birds with one biscuit, if you will. (Thank you, Justin Bilancieri, for the bird-friendly twist on an old saying.)

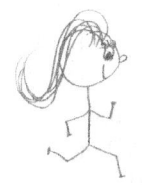

A Complicated Case of Incontinence with Running

Because so many of my patients specifically seek therapy when they cannot run without leaking, I am revisiting the topic to stress the importance of finding and addressing every aspect of the problem. As I mentioned previously, a low body temperature and a high level of cortisol may trigger urinary urgency. But, some cases of urgency upon running just after emptying a very full bladder may not be due to cortisol's alleged stimulatory effect. Weakness, fatigue, and incomplete voiding may come into play and need to be addressed to resolve incontinence with running.

As I explained in an earlier section entitled *'Incomplete Voiding'*, urgency to revisit the restroom after having just emptied a full bladder may be due to backlogged urine trickling into the bladder after the bladder is emptied, but while the bladder is still in *'go mode'*. This happens when the bladder becomes so full the amount of urine collected cannot fit in the bladder and collects in the ureters until space becomes available in the bladder. If the bladder is indeed full initially, the ureters pour urine into the bladder when the bladder is still in *'go mode'*, like the cars entering the freeway from the onramps, as soon as space becomes available. Exercise that jolts the body may quicken the flow of backlogged urine out of the ureters and into the newly emptied bladder. It is quite common to use the restroom before setting out to run. If urine had backlogged in the ureters, the jolt of running could hasten its entry into the bladder while the body is still in *'go mode'*, and the runner may experience urgency. The urge may strike as early as a few steps into the route or as late as 15 minutes into hitting the trail. Upon stopping to void, the runner may find that the amount of urine is minimal. Kegeling can curb this urge (to purge, haha!) if the pelvic floor muscles are strong enough to pulse messages to the brain's micturition center to halt the detrusor's contraction via the feedback loop. The stronger the pelvic floor's contraction, the more effective the feedback is in controlling this urge.

But, what about a sudden onset of extreme urgency after running 20-30 minutes? Such was the case for 37 year-old Casey, who experienced urinary urgency, stress urinary incontinence (especially when sneezing and running), and incomplete void. Casey's condition came on suddenly when she noted that she could not hold the urine stream after running for 30 minutes. (Note, previous cases with a possible cortisol effect stressed the difficulty contracting against urges at the outset of running. This case was quite the opposite.) Casey also noted strong urgency upon approaching a restroom, as with the *key in the door syndrome*, and strong urgency even minutes after having just voided. With such urgency after having just voided, urinary frequency was also an issue. The common denominator was an overly exerted, under-rested pelvic floor, which was already weakened by a disadvantageous length-tension relationship born of right ilial (side of pelvis) elevation.

Casey had a difficult time fully voiding, noting dribbling and a need to void after standing from toilet. She also reported difficulty contracting the pelvic floor in isolation for more than three seconds, after which she would incorporate the abdominals. Such abdominal contraction, as previously stated, can enhance urgency and overly work the pelvic floor muscles when attempting to counter the urge. Consequently, the actual ability to contract the pelvic floor was not Casey's biggest issue. Rather, it was the inability to fully relax, like in Anna's case, which resulted in an overly fatigued pelvic floor. The ilial asymmetry did contribute to the weakness, as Casey noted a stronger contraction with alignment. But the greatest gains were made once Casey could fully relax. As soon as Casey could fully release the pelvic floor, she was able to fully void and she noted a vast improvement in contraction. With the pelvic floor no longer overly fatigued, she was able to contract strongly enough to curb the urge and counter the stress of a sneeze.

To get a bit technical…As in Anna's case, Casey's pelvic floor muscles had been overly exerted with a constant contraction. Constant contraction disallowed full voiding as the micturition center was signaled to hold the urine with detrusor inhibition. With fatigue of the pelvic floor muscles, however, the micturition center would disinhibit the detrusor and a strong sense of urinary urgency would ensue. The vicious cycle grew out of too strong of a contraction when the pelvic floor was to be relaxed, and too feeble of a contraction to control an urge! The fatigue on top of the overly lengthened muscle fibers also disallowed the strong burst of contraction needed to counter the intra-abdominal pressure added with a cough or a sneeze.

Casey's difficulty holding after running 30 minutes likely stemmed from a baseline of fatiguing tension at the beginning of the run. The pelvic floor muscles were too tense to fully relax and allow for the bladder to completely empty before the run. This constant state of tension also likely fatigued the pelvic floor muscles, and when an urge developed from the previous incomplete void, she eventually became too fatigued to counter it. Adding intra-abdominal pressure with running's jolt likely worsened the urge. In such a fatigued state, the pelvic floor likely did not have enough energy to pulse messages to the micturition center to inhibit the bladder's detrusor contraction after 30 minutes. Urgency then developed, with a subsequent need to void. The vicious, incontinent cycle recurred with successive attempts at running.

The main focus of Casey's therapy was to regain control of the pelvic floor so as to first relax the pelvic floor muscles, and then contract them in isolation. Casey responded very well to the *lava flow* exercise aimed at relaxing the pelvic floor. While sitting on a large therapy ball, she Kegeled first, then blew through pursed lips while concentrating on relaxing the pelvic floor. Exhaling while sitting on the ball, she could feel a pressure change in the perineum (undersurface of her groin) like lava flowing slowly down a volcano. Initially she needed to exhale 3 times in a row before fully relaxing. After a few attempts, though, she was able to fully relax after 2 exhalations. After the very first visit, instead of sensing fatigue with repeated pelvic floor contractions, Casey noted a stronger ability to isolate the contraction as relaxation between each Kegel attempt was achieved.

To add a little more spice to the mix, the number of Casey's episodes of stress urinary incontinence increased pre-menstrually. As previously stated, there is a pre-menstrual surge of estrogen,[20] and elevated estrogen levels have been found to associate with a higher incidence of incontinence.[19] In addition, water retention often experienced during that time increased pressure within Casey's pelvic region. Such a baseline of pressure can place greater demands on the pelvic floor. When Casey's pelvic floor muscles were already countering pressure caused by water retention and potentially adversely affected by estrogen, a sneeze's burst of intra-abdominal pressure had a greater chance of breaking the pelvic floor's holding power... hence her heightened incidence of premenstrual stress urinary incontinence.

Many aspects of a woman's life can interfere with continence, as depicted in Casey's case. Extra Kegels pre-menstrually can reinforce the contraction needed to counter stress urinary incontinence, should estrogen potentiate a spike in its incidence. Improving Kegel strength can also help counter extra pressure experienced with pelvic water retention. I explained to Casey the normalcy of occurrences that can interfere with continence. This education helped Casey to proactively prepare with extra pelvic floor activation pre-menstrually. It also motivated her to practice the contract/relax *lava flow* exercises to ensure her pelvic floor muscles had enough energy to counter incontinence while on a premenstrual run! (See Figure 26.)

Figure 26. An example of an evaluation of a patient presenting with mixed incontinence due to overly fatigued and guarded pelvic floor muscles.

Diagnoses: Complicated case of mixed incontinence and incomplete void, with right ilial elevation

Upon evaluation, the following were noted:
1. Patient reports onset of stress urinary incontinence, urinary urgency, and incomplete void leading to frequency with the birth of her child 10/16/06.
2. Patient particularly notes strong, uncontrollable urgency after ~ 30 minutes of running.
3. Right ilial elevation correlates with tension in right greater than left lumbar paraspinals, and with mechanics of habitually carrying child on right with right ilium elevated.
4. Pt reports difficulty relaxing the pelvic floor muscles, taking 3 steps to release.
5. With the pelvic floor muscles overly contracting in a guarded state, they are likely too fatigued to contract and endure a strong hold.
6. The guarding correlates with difficulty releasing and incomplete void.
7. Full relaxation is likely needed in order for muscle fatigue to resolve. With resolution of muscle fatigue, full contraction will likely be achieved.
8. With ilial alignment, patient's ease of contraction and relaxation of pelvic floor increased by ~ 30%.
9. Lumbar-pelvic stabilization is recommended, however, we will commence with isolated pelvic floor contractions. Currently the patient is able to contract the pelvic floor in isolation of the abdominals, albeit weakly, but only with highly concentrated effort. Once the isolation of the pelvic floor is second nature, we will commence full core exercises.
10. With estrogen surges pre-menstrually and/or added pressure of water retention pre-menstrually, difficulty holding the pelvic floor muscles is not unexpected.
11. Should electrical stimulation and/or electrical biofeedback be appropriate and necessary, measures will be taken.

Plan/Goals:
1. Independent with home exercise program.
2. Isolation of pelvic floor muscle contraction.
3. Ilial symmetry held with home exercises.
4. Independent timing of the pelvic floor to counter incontinence.
5. Full void and pelvic floor relaxation.
6. No episodes of incontinence.

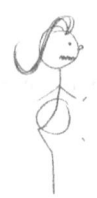

Pregnancy and Incontinence

Pregnancy can exert enormous pressures on the bladder and induce strain within the pelvic cavity, setting the pelvic floor muscles up for failure against incontinence. To fit a growing uterus in the pelvic cavity, the ligaments that hold the pelvic bones in place may relax to allow for the pelvis to expand.[14] This laxity can come at a cost if it associates with pelvic asymmetry, such as an upward shift and/or a rotation on one side of the pelvis relative to the other. (See previous Figures 7a, 7b, 8, 10a, and 10b.) These asymmetries can cause disadvantageous over-lengthening of the pelvic floor muscle fibers, weakening their holding power against incontinence. In addition, carrying another human in the uterus adds to the pelvic floor's burden of keeping all the contents of the pelvic cavity in place! Overly worked and possibly overly lengthened, the pelvic floor's muscle fibers may not be in top shape to counter incontinence on multiple fronts during pregnancy.

Pregnancy is often associated with stress urinary incontinence for the obvious reason of an enlarged and heavy uterus pressing on the bladder. A growing uterus can create a progressively stronger force on the bladder. This force can simulate that of the bladder's detrusor muscle contracting to void, but with a weight on top. To put this in perspective, allow me to use the previously described hose metaphor: Think about trying to squeeze a hose shut with a fist while water flows through the hose at full speed. Then imagine a heavy rock dropping onto the hose a few inches from your fist. The added pressure of the rock would definitely make the hose harder to hold shut!

Urinary frequency is common with pregnancy. The excessive physical pressure exerted on the bladder by the growing uterus can push on the internal sphincter and mimic a heavy, full bladder even if the bladder is not even half full. This pressure on the sphincter can create urinary urgency that, when weakly combatted by fatigued and weakened pelvic floor muscles, can lead to urinary frequency.

During pregnancy, the weight of the uterus can also induce a mechanical change whereby both sides of the pelvic sit in an anterior or forward tilt. The relaxin hormone released during pregnancy acts as an accomplice to the pelvic movement with its enhancement of ligamentous laxity.[14] The anterior (forward) rotation of the pelvis often leads to hyperlordosis, or sway back, with ensuing foraminal encroachment on neural structures. With this narrowed pathway, the nerves can become irritated. Irritation inflames the nerves, making them larger than normal. The enlarged nerve can be further compressed in its narrowing pathway, leading to more irritation, and more inflammation. (See Figure 27.) The encroachment may lead to pain and to inadequate function. Pelvic floor weakness may result from cranky, uncooperative sacral nerves. The pelvic floor cannot afford weakness, especially while attempting to counter the weight of a growing uterus pressing on the bladder. Physical therapy can help to correct the hyperlordosis (sway back) by strengthening the abdominals and resolving any tension in the low back muscles that would pull the spine into excessive lordosis. Reducing the lordosis, or sway, can open the pathways for the nerves to travel. Once relieved, the nerves can resume normal stimulation to the muscles with appropriate physical therapy. With sufficient implementation of the Kegel into daily activities, continence can be restored.[34]

Figure 27. Illustration of a hyperlordotic spine with narrow neural pathways compared to a neutral spine with adequately spaced neural pathways.

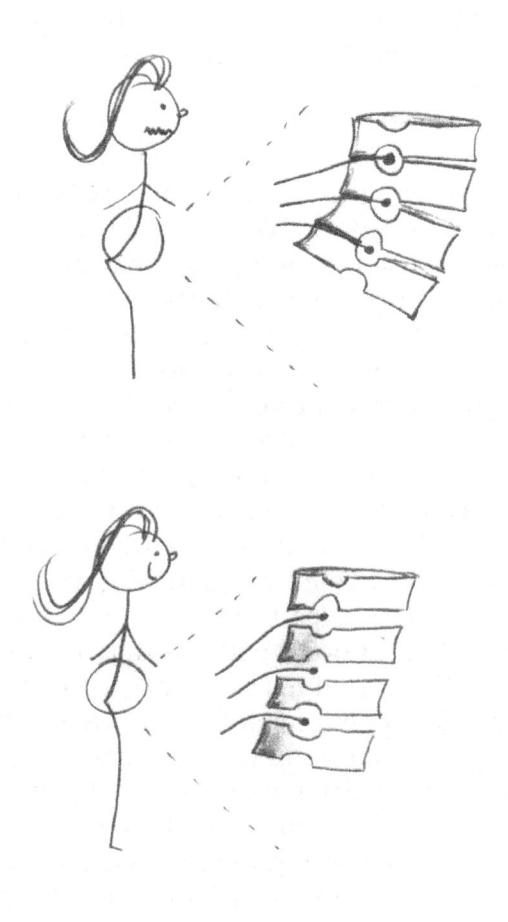

In addition to hyperlordosis, or sway back, the relaxin-induced ligament laxity may also cause malalignment of the sacroiliac joints along the backside of the pelvic cavity. Like ilial (pelvic) obliquities, the sacroiliac joint asymmetries can often lead to incontinence. The previously described ilial (pelvic) flares and rotations and sacral flares may emerge as causes of the pelvic floor's dysfunction. In these cases, the sacral nerves *and* the pelvic floor muscles are vulnerable to skewing out of their normal anatomical array. Weakness may arise out of irritated nerves *and* altered muscle fiber length-tension relationships. Treatments to optimize the neural and muscular integrity must be integrated into the treatments to resolve incontinence. Otherwise, the sources of the stress urinary incontinence, urgency, and frequency would be left to fester.

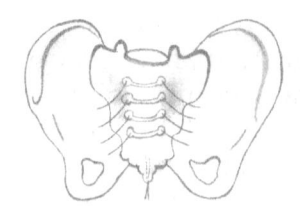

Childbirth and Incontinence

Pregnancy is a common instigator, but women often face incontinence *after* childbirth. Trauma of childbirth takes the pelvic floor muscles fatigued from a 9-month long marathon hold, and inflames them. The inflammation on top of the fatigue can make the muscles even less likely to cooperate. Women with incontinence after childbirth may be able to perform a contraction of the pelvic floor, but it is often weak and low in endurance. Childbirth may also move the sacroiliac joints and ilia (sides of pelvis) out of alignment, disrupting neural pathways and causing a disadvantageous length-tension relationship among the pelvic floor's muscle fibers. Sadly, with any and all of the above, incontinence is often born alongside the child.

Trauma to the vaginal walls with childbirth is often a hefty cause for incontinence. Muscle guarding, nerve damage, and overly lengthened pelvic floor muscle fibers all may contribute to inadequate control over urine flow. Muscle guarding in the pelvic region may emerge in conjunction with the trauma of childbirth, as it can in the calf muscle with a trauma to the leg. The guarded muscles hold in a protective state. With the potential consequence of fatigue, the pelvic floor often has difficulty *strongly* contracting when a sneeze or cough approaches. Its guarded state can also create a roadblock when attempting to *fully relax* to void. The trauma of childbirth, then, can very well birth stress urinary incontinence, incomplete voiding, urinary urgency, and urinary frequency.

After childbirth, the way a mother carries her child may potentially perpetuate incontinence. A woman commonly carries her child on one side of her pelvis, with that ilium in an elevated position. (See previous Figure 8.) This elevated ilial position is a leading cause of a disadvantageously lengthened and weakened pelvic floor. With successive pregnancies, a mother may be carrying one child on an elevated ilium while carrying another in the womb. Elevation of the ilium and pregnancy each separately predispose incontinence. Together, the effects of both may result in a higher probability of excessive muscle fatigue, urinary leakage, urinary urgency, and urinary frequency.

Even if the best ergonomics are utilized, lifting and carrying a child both increase intra-abdominal pressure. This intra-abdominal pressure pushes on the bladder, increasing the demand on the pelvic floor muscles to counter urine flow. Carrying the child on the hip with the pelvis asymmetrically elevated can weaken the pelvic floor muscle fibers. These two scenarios each can tax the pelvic floor individually; together the burden often leads to pelvic floor muscle failure.

Adding fuel to the incontinent fire…I have come across many a patient who experience difficulty sensing the urine flow, especially after multiple childbirths. Reduced sensation often disallows engagement of the voluntary contraction to counter the flow out of the urethra. When the stretch reflex in the bladder's detrusor muscle is alive and well, and urine flows without the patient's awareness, leaking may be inevitable.

Rehabilitation with a timed voiding schedule can help to regain control over emptying the bladder voluntarily instead of involuntarily and uncontrollably. Over time, as the patient develops more control over voluntarily contracting the pelvic floor, a heightened awareness of urine in the urinary pathway can develop. There seems to be a sensory awakening that occurs with the improvement in pelvic floor control.

In summary, for many of my patients, physical therapy helps fight incontinence after childbirth by dispelling its causes and strategically implementing exercises to restore pelvic floor muscle strength and agility. The incontinence after childbirth often appears to stem from an accumulation of physical stress and a disadvantageous array of pelvic floor muscle fibers, each presenting alone or in cahoots. Inadequate muscle strength and poor timing can be especially problematic when patients have a weak or nonexistent sensation of urine flow. Mechanics training to appropriately hold and carry a child is usually one aspect of the therapy. Ilial (pelvic) alignment is often another. The reacquisition of pelvic floor control and sensation in the urinary pathway is usually achieved with guided exercise, sometimes accompanied by electrical vaginal stimulation. Full core training can follow pelvic floor isolation training. Once again, it is important to isolate the pelvic floor muscles first, as this improves upon incontinence. Full core training should be integrated for lumbar-pelvic support after successful pelvic floor isolation is achieved. The core's grip on the pelvic region can minimize the recurrence of ilial (pelvic) asymmetries and thusly optimize the newly reacquired pelvic floor muscle integrity.

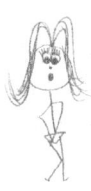

Two to Four Weeks into Rehabilitation And a Regression Rears??

I have encountered a common occurrence with my patients after two to four weeks of therapy, at which time a significant regression spontaneously occurs. The patients can often isolate the pelvic floor, counter small amounts of intra-abdominal pressure, and incorporate the timing of the contractions to curb a light urge. Then, seemingly out of nowhere, the patients are socked with regression and temporarily leak uncontrollably.

Why the abrupt regression? As of the publication of this book, I was unable to find research supporting explanations, but there are a couple that make sense. A 'rebooting' of the neural pathways is one possible answer. The feedback loop and/or neural pathways associated with a voluntary contraction may essentially become overloaded and need a chance to 'reset'. Another possible answer involves estrogen's potential contribution to incontinence. As discussed previously, estrogen levels elevate at ovulation and premenstrually.[20] Some patients may not be strong enough Kegel-wise to combat estrogen's potential effect of making urine control more challenging. The good news is that this regression is usually only temporary. After 3-5 days, progress usually emerges again, and the patients are back on track. If a premenstrual regression recurs, it is most often not nearly as dramatic as the regression 2-4 weeks into therapy. As long as strength and agility gains are progressively made, the recurrent regression is usually minimal. At times, the patient may temporarily find it more difficult to contract the pelvic floor muscles, but another abrupt halt in control is not common.

Upon her second visit, Sarah presented with ilial alignment, resolution of low back and pelvic pain, and she reported greater ease contracting the pelvic floor musculature. Upon her third visit, ilial alignment and painfree status continued, however she noted a marked regression in pelvic floor contraction! Visit three occurred two weeks after her initial visit and coincidentally just before commencement of her menses. Was the regression due to the hypothetical resetting of the feedback loop? Or, was the premenstrual estrogen surge responsible for the regression? In either case, gains in length of tetanic Kegel hold resumed upon her fourth visit, which coincided with the cessation of her menses.

The regression at the 2-4 week mark is so common, I tell nearly all of my patients at the start of therapy. I do not want to encourage patients to create a self-fulfilling prophecy, but I do want to enlighten them on the intricate nature of pelvic floor control. Furthermore, knowing ahead of time, patients can plan for the unexpected. If a patient has made enough headway to only need one undergarment per day, the regression may require 2 or 3. This is especially helpful if the patient is going on a trip ~ 2-4 weeks after the start of therapy to a place where undergarments are hard to come by! Knowledge is power. Being apprised of the potential regression can help the patient not only prepare in a practical sense for the possible increase in leaking, it can prepare the patient mentally with the understanding that the potential decrease in control is only temporary, keeping her motivated to continue her conquest for continence.

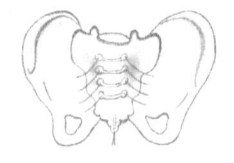

Space Invaders…

The *'celes*, as I like to call prolapses, are the space invaders that often trigger stress urinary incontinence. These protrusions into the vaginal walls may alter the positioning of the urethra and overstretch the walls of the vagina, both of which disrupt the pelvic floor's ability to hold strongly against incontinence.

To detect the protrusions, ultrasound and evacuation proctography can be used to visually depict the contours of the 'celes in the pelvic cavity.[35,36] Some research shows, however, that protrusions are best detected with clinical assessments.[37] However detected, the protrusions are named according to their origins. The falling of the bladder is known as a bladder prolapse or cystocele. A urethrocele is a falling of the urethra into the vagina. Protrusion resulting from the falling of the rectum is a rectal prolapse or rectocele. An enterocele results from the small bowel's protrusion into the anterior (front) of the vagina.[7] Childbirth often results in a prolapse of the vaginal walls into themselves due to overstretching.[6,7] Such a protrusion is termed a vaginocele or colpocele.[38] A prolapse of the uterus can cause a protrusion of the vagina into the itself,[6,7] thereby causing a vaginocele. The 'celes disrupt the normal team approach to holding the organs in place, the team members being the pelvic floor and the mesh of tissue surrounding the organs. The mesh and the pelvic floor ordinarily act together as a cargo net. With the protrusions, the supportive net may begin to unravel and the pelvic floor's muscle fibers may disadvantageously lengthen. The pelvic floor muscles may struggle to hold tight, with the task of holding the fallen structures and the urine stream difficult if not impossible.

"My insides are falling out!"

For the 'celes I have encountered clinically, Kegels can assist in holding the contents of the pelvic cavity stable. A study showed that Kegel exercises are crucial to successful continence in patients with cystocele, and greatly assist in alleviating a cystocele's associated low back pain. Organ displacement can create a painful state in the low back and pelvic region. Further pain can emerge from muscle guarding. Pressures on the intra-abdominal fascia and abdominal walls can create a state of instability and wreak painful havoc. Holding the pelvic floor muscles can create a state of stability and support, rendering relief from pain.[39]

The 'celes require extra care to restore the functional capacity of the pelvic floor musculature *without* over-fatiguing. Fatigue can lead to a sensation of heaviness or a feeling that organs are pushing downward, as was the case for Kim after having twins. This sensation represents a pushing of the prolapses against other organs, i.e. the uterus pushing into the vagina and against the vaginal walls. Contracting the pelvic floor can reduce such sensation of heaviness, likely due to the lifting of the undersurface that serves as a base on which the organs sit. The symmetry of the pelvis is important to maximize the efficiency of the pelvic floor, as described previously in the section entitled *'Asymmetries Often Underlie a Mechanical Disadvantage of the Pelvic Floor'*. (See previous

Figures 7a-11.) If the pelvic floor is over-fatigued, not only is incontinence imminent, the organs are also on the brink of falling into or through the vagina! Communication between the patient and clinician is a crucial part of the game plan to strengthen smartly and effectively.

But, wait! What about the pelvic floor musculature that is working on overdrive as a sole core supporter to compensate for weak deep abdominal musculature? Several patients with the 'celes have found remarkable success with deep abdominal strengthening. I have had a number of patients with one or more of the 'celes report considerably less "heaviness" and less of a sensation that their "insides are falling out" as they improved upon pulling their navel to their spine to strengthen the transverse abdominis...even with the most rigorous of activity! Why? As previously discussed in the section entitled *'Weakened Abdominal Musculature and a Tie to Stress Urinary Incontinence'*, the pelvic floor may overly exert in trying to hold the spine and pelvis stable without the assistance of the transverse abdominis, all the while acting as a platform for the pelvic organs. Once the transverse abdominis regains strength, the pelvic floor can shed a good deal of its burden of supporting the bony structures. With strong deep abdominal support, the pelvic floor does not have to work as hard on a daily basis, and can thus rejuvenate. This renewal of energy in the pelvic floor muscles can give the pelvic organs the floor support they need to remain intact, and the patients can resume their rigorous lives with greater confidence that their "insides" will remain inside!

In some cases of prolapse, a mesh sling is surgically implanted to hold the bladder, uterus, and other pelvic contents in their appropriate positions. The sling can also hold the urethra stable to keep the internal sphincter from opening inappropriately. The mesh sling is secured internally connecting from the proximal urethra, to the pelvic floor, to the rectus fascia,[40] acting as a safety net per se. I find that the sling is more effective, however, with assistance from the pelvic floor muscles when intra-abdominal pressures abound. With such pressure, the sling can overstretch, and potentially fail. The struggling sling can mimic an overstretched ligament failing to keep a joint intact. Without the backing of strong, agile, and well-timed muscle contractions, the sling, like an overstretched ligament barely supporting a joint, can fail to keep the pelvic floor contents in position. Therefore, even with sling support, strong pelvic floor musculature is integral to continence, organ support, and pain cessation.

Abdominal Exercise Amidst Pelvic Floor Training

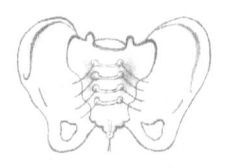

Abdominal Exercise and Overcoming Incontinence

Is It Possible to Exercise the Abdominal Muscles En Route to Conquering Incontinence?

Yes, it is...but in due time. The ability to resume an abdominal workout is dependent on Kegel timing and strength! Once the isolation of the pelvic floor contraction is achieved and gains are made in curbing incontinence, performing an abdominal workout may not be counterproductive to gaining continence. However, adding an abdominal exercise regime does *not* bode well for the patient who fails to isolate the pelvic floor and fails to hold the pelvic floor contraction against added intra-abdominal pressure. Abdominal exercise increases the pressure on the bladder, which in turn increases the chances of incontinence. The intra-abdominal pressure increases with an abdominal workout just it would with coughing, sneezing, laughing, lifting, jumping, carrying, and running. The patient should be able to isolate the pelvic floor from the abdominals and time the Kegel around applied intra-abdominal pressure in order to hold continent with an abdominal workout. Let's use a plank as an example of an abdominal exercise. Successfully holding continent while performing a plank requires contracting the pelvic floor muscles in isolation first, holding that contraction throughout the plank, finishing the plank, *then* releasing the pelvic floor muscle contraction. If the patient cannot isolate *and* hold the pelvic floor contraction against added intra-abdominal pressure, she risks leaking when performing the plank. Therefore, abdominal workouts should only be added when the patient is indeed making gains toward continence with activities that add intra-abdominal pressure.

In a sense, when I am training patients to counter intra-abdominal pressure, I am asking the patients to contract the abdominals, but not in a conscious manner. The timing exercises with lifting, pressing on a therapy ball, stepping up and down a step, transferring position, catching and throwing a ball, and pulling and pushing a cord all incorporate use of the abdominals. However, the patient's focus is on Kegeling around the activity and not on the abdominal activation.

Though the abdominal contraction with these simulations and activities is not conscious, it does indeed add intra-abdominal pressure as an abdominal workout would. The difference with an abdominal workout, however, is that the abdominal contraction is a conscious effort, taking focus away from the pelvic floor. Just like training a patient to contract the full core for pelvic stabilization, I make sure the patient understands that it is imperative to contract the pelvic floor around the abdominal contraction. To keep pelvic floor control in the foreground, the Kegel must be performed and held while performing the abdominal exercise and the Kegel must be released only after completion of the abdominal contraction.

Once isolated contractions begin to curb incontinence, patients eager to exercise the abdominals are instructed to begin with short intervals of abdominal contractions. I may recommend starting with a plank in a diagonal position for 5 seconds, of course with the Kegel timing in check. The patient may then increase the number of repetitions as long as she is able to hold the Kegel throughout each plank. If the pelvic floor muscles fatigue, it is time to take a break. After 1-2 minutes, another round of the planking may begin. As appropriate, the patient may progress to 10-second holds in a diagonal position, then to 10-second holds in a horizontal position. The numbers of repetitions and sets build in accordance with the ability to Kegel around the planks. This way, the patient does not lose sight of pelvic floor control, but is able to resume an abdominal workout.

I have found it helpful for the patients to think of themselves as two separate patients when Kegeling to counter urine flow and Kegeling in conjunction with an abdominal exercise. One performs Kegels in isolation of an unconsciously added abdominal contraction to counter urine flow and the other Kegels around the consciously afforded abdominal contraction when performing an abdominal workout. This may initially seem contradictory to a holistic approach, but it works! The timing of the isolated contraction to counter incontinence is reinforced, and confusion as to when the abdominal muscles are allowed to contract is avoided.

Abdominal control is crucial to trunk control and postural strength. Keeping a strong abdominal section balances the pull of the dorsal (back) muscles. The abdominals work with the back muscles to hold the spine in a comfortable and healthy neutral position. With proper timing, the abdominals can be conditioned to keep the trunk healthy without compromising the pursuit of continence.

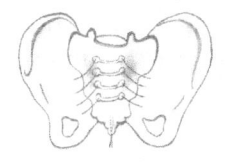

Abdominal Exercise and Prolapse

Is It Possible to Exercise Abdominal Muscles En Route to Conquering a Prolapse?

Exercising the abdominals while fighting a prolapse is tricky. Adding abdominal pressure can make it difficult to hold the pelvic floor to support the contents of the abdominal cavity. As previously emphasized, a healthy and balanced trunk is needed for stabilization of the spine and pelvis, especially when lifting, carrying, walking, and changing position. It is also very important to keep the pelvic contents contained.

Once the pelvic floor can counter the added intra-abdominal force, the patient can begin abdominal exercise in the supine, quadruped, or plank position. The timing of the Kegel and the ability to sustain the Kegel throughout the abdominal exercise is paramount to keeping the pelvic contents secure. It is important to remember that countering the abdominal exercise can fatigue the pelvic floor, which is already being taxed by a falling organ. High endurance is necessary to sustain the positional integrity of the pelvic contents with the abdominal exercise *and thereafter* with the rest of the day's activities. It is important to be mindful of the whereabouts of the pelvic contents, keeping in mind that an increase in pressure in the pelvic region can be a signal that an organ is falling. If the prolapse is worsening, the patient should halt the abdominal exercise until the prolapse is controlled, then resume with an interval regime that suits the pelvic floor's endurance level.

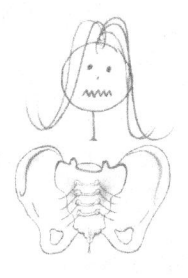

Pelvic Pain

An excellent question perplexed Cece, one of my patients with pelvic pain: Why does the body not heal itself from childbirth or trauma over the course of time? Cece posed this question after giving birth to five children, sustaining a motor vehicle accident after the birth of her third child, and falling off of a quad bike onto her right side, fracturing her tailbone. My answer? Multiple traumas without adequate recovery time can hinder healing....and a darn good physical therapist could be helpful!

In response to trauma, the body's tissues may release bradykinins, prostaglandins, and histamine. These chemicals swarm to protect the damaged region, and swelling develops.[41] With time, strengthening, and good circulation, these chemicals can be removed. With multiple traumas, however, these chemicals may be repeatedly produced and the swelling can persist.[42] The presence of lingering inflammatory products seems to create painful tension in the tissues. For my patients who have sustained such traumas, manual therapy (similar to massage) has helped to move the chemicals out of their affected tissues, thereby reducing the swelling, and reducing the pain. Strengthening can help to rebuild the infrastructure encasing the affected region. This boost of support to the recovering regions can tell the body's inflammation factory to halt production. Restoring mobility and strength (and appropriate alignment if applicable) can help resolve painful tension and send the patient down the road to recovery.

If repeated use and strain with daily activities outweigh recovery, the tissues are susceptible to repeated inflammatory responses and to further and further breakdown. Repetitive strains with inadequate recovery often inflict rotator cuff lesions and patellar tendinitis. The same repetitive strain phenomenon occurs across the pelvis as was clearly depicted by the aforementioned multiple birth and trauma scenario. Multiple births, falling and fracturing the tailbone, straining with a motor vehicle accident, and further straining while holding a child on one side of the pelvis in a hiked or elevated position all together create an onslaught of repetitive strain. Multiple feedings that minimize can usurp recovery time. Awkward positioning can disrupt Mom's recovery during actual sleep time if her little children crawl into her bed. Awkward positioning can perpetuate the strain, and therefore impede healing. With all strain and minimal recovery, a scenario of bodily breakdown can precipitate a trip to physical therapy.

In my many years of experience, I have seen strengthening keep the small traumas from creating a recurring inflammatory response. With good conditioning, the tissues are supported and have what I like to call a *recovery memory*. Bodily tissues break down with exercise, and with rest the tissues can recover and strengthen. If another trauma occurs before recovering from the previous one, fatigue and pain may set it, and swelling may occur. The stronger the tissues, the better they seem to be at recovering. Better recovery can minimize inflammation with daily micro-traumas. Thus, exercise can teach the body to break down and recover, recover being the operative word. The better the recovery rate, the better the body may be at overcoming the strains life's activities throw its way.

According to a 1995 study, pelvic pain may also associate with high levels of relaxin hormone which has been found in pregnant and nonpregnant women with pelvic pain.[43] Some studies show an association of serum levels of relaxin and pelvic pain, with the inherent nature of relaxin creating ligamentous laxity.[34] The instability associated with ligaments' laxity may contribute to joint pain, muscle guarding, and ilial (pelvic) obliquities. Throughout the human body, ligamentous laxity can result in a reliance on muscle activity for the support of joint structures. Muscles *can* be trained to *actively* support bony joints, the key word being "actively". Ligaments are designed to support without a lag in time, however the muscles that are compensating for their laxity do have a lag time in that time is needed for the muscles to react to a destabilizing occurrence. Strength and especially agility training are chief means of effectively stabilizing the joints, minimizing associated pain.

Trauma and pelvic joint instability can lead to excessive muscle tension or guarding in the pelvic floor. The guarded musculature can bring pain and cramping to the abdominal cavity. Guarding can rear untimely contraction of the pelvic floor muscles when attempting to fully void as it can cause painful tension during intercourse. In a previous section entitled *'Pelvic Floor Relaxation as Rehabilitation's Driving Force'*, muscle guarding was blamed for overly fatiguing the pelvic floor in patients, such as Mandy, Anna, and Casey, and leading to episodes of incontinence. Guarding, therefore, can wreak havoc threefold provoking incomplete void, painful intercourse, and incontinence. Hip flexor and hip rotator muscle tension may accompany pelvic floor guarding, and should not be overlooked. Releasing the tension and showing the patient how to do so can help to resolve these conditions and minimize their recurrence. (See Figures 28-30.) Treating the underlying cause of the tension and building control of the pelvic floor muscles can complement the tension release, which can ultimately assist in resolving the pain associated with pelvic dysfunction.

Figure 28. Stretching to release tension in the iliopsoas (hip flexor) muscle.

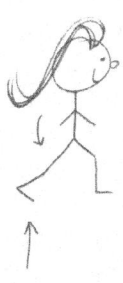

Figure 29. Stretching to release muscle tension in the hip's internal rotators.

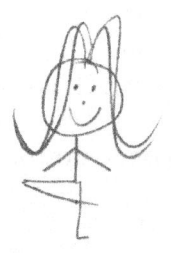

Figure 30. Stretching to release tension in the hip's external rotator muscles.

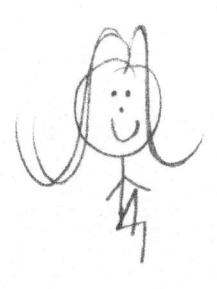

Sitting gently on a soft, sand filled medicine ball can alleviate painful tension in the pelvic floor muscles. Fitting the pliable ball between the vagina and the anus gently adds pressure to the superficial layers of the pelvic floor musculature. Patients should be in control of the amount of pressure exerted, making this technique a self-administered, gentle compression massage. (See Figure 31). The idea of adding pressure to release pressure can work to release the tension in the targeted muscles. With tension release, pain usually reduces. With repetitive sessions of pressure release and pain reduction, the inflammation that had occurred in response to pain can gradually reduce, then cease when the pain has resolved. Resolution of the inflammation can continue as control over the pelvic floor muscles builds. Similar to conditioning the arms and legs, exercise can teach the pelvic floor muscles to contract *and* relax, and a normalized resting tone can develop. Isolated, well-timed Kegels can normalize the resting tone of the pelvic floor, revive strong contractions to counter incontinence, and help restore the ability to adequately release the pelvic floor muscles to void and rest.

Figure 31. Gently sitting on a soft medicine ball to release tension in the pelvic floor muscles.

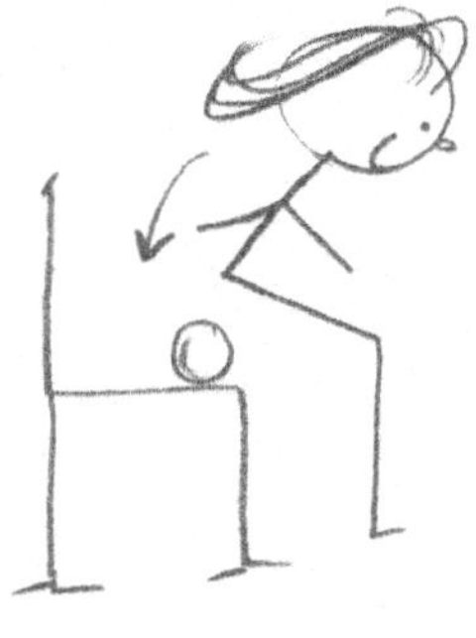

In conjunction with the self-administered pressure release trick with the medicine ball, reverse Kegels or conscious relaxations of the pelvic floor muscles with the *lava flow* exercises can provide a means to soften the tension, ease full void, and alleviate pain with intercourse. The *blow when you go* technique can help! Repeatedly blowing through pursed lips as when attempting to fully void can provide a means of fully relaxing. After the first blow, the patient may *think* she is relaxed because relative to her previously tense state, she is! To her surprise, however, muscle guarding and tension often need a second or even a third try in order to release. Sequential releases while sitting on the small ball (for muscle decompression) can ultimately result in pelvic floor muscle relaxation.

The small medicine ball can also be used to test the level of pain harnessed within the pelvic floor muscles. The irritability spectrum spans from an inability to sit due to pain to sitting comfortably on the ball with full pressure. Because pain tolerance, body weight, and general like or dislike of pressure release massage can vary from person to person, using the ball to determine the irritability level of the pelvic floor muscles is a patient specific, subjective test. With successive treatments to help relax the pelvic floor muscles, the tolerance to the pressure of sitting on the small ball usually builds. A greater ability to sit on the ball and a more favorable response to the pressure usually correlate with greater success in fully voiding and less overall pain with daily activity.

Sitting on a large therapy ball and performing the previously described *lava flow* exercise can help patients sense when they are relaxing the pelvic floor muscles. As mentioned, there is a tactile sensation of light pressure around the perineum whilst sitting on the ball. With relaxation, the sensation moves downward and outward like lava flowing down a volcano. This *lava flow* exercise helps patients to sense where they are to be relaxing and when they have fully released. The *lava flow* exercise can ultimately assist in reducing excessive habitual tension and pain.

Initially Olivia presented with such tension in the perineal muscles, and sitting on a soft medicine ball on the first visit was out of the question. After 3 weeks of intermittently contracting the pelvic floor with a Kegel, then relaxing the pelvic floor with a *blow when you go* exercise, the tension in the perineum dropped to where Olivia was able to fully sit on the soft medicine ball without pain. This translated into fully voiding and resolution of pain with intercourse.

When trying to increase the voluntary control of painful pelvic floor muscles, the Kegel contraction itself can increase pain. I have often found this to be the case when the coccyx (or tailbone) is unstable and when the guarding of the pelvic floor is so intense that further contraction is too painful to perform. A heavily guarded pelvic floor can pull too strongly on the coccyx (tailbone), creating a state of pain. Releasing the pelvic floor muscles can allow for appropriate repositioning of the tailbone. A gradual increase in pelvic floor control can then hold the coccyx (tailbone) stable in its correct position without pulling too harshly. Hip and pelvic muscles alongside those of the pelvic floor can also pull on the coccyx (tailbone) or on the fascia (connective tissue) attaching to it. Releasing tension in the hip rotators and low back muscles can resolve the excess pull, further resolving the pain with the Kegel contraction. (See previous Figures 16a, 16b, 29 and 30.) The coccygeal (tailbone) pain can resolve with greater stability in its appropriate position, and stability can be achieved with greater pelvic floor control. A gradual progression from short, gentle Kegels to longer, yet gentle, Kegels can start to enhance the patient's control over the pelvic floor, and start to stabilize the coccyx and resolve the coccygeal pain. With improvements in coccygeal stability and pain resolution, the strength of the Kegel can increase, promoting continued improvements in overall pelvic floor control.

For patients with intense pelvic floor muscle guarding who cannot Kegel due to muscle pain, Kegeling while standing with hips abducted or with feet apart can work wonders! Although it is often difficult to hold against urine flow in this position because of a longer distance the muscle fibers have to slide in order to close the external sphincter, there may be less painful tension on the guarded muscles. Reducing the pain in the pelvic floor muscles can allow the patients to Kegel with less pain so they can start to regain control over the pelvic floor, as I will explain with Rita's case.

Initially Rita presented with painful tension in the pelvic floor muscles, and contracting the pelvic floor increased that pain. Sitting on a soft medicine ball on the first visit was out of the question. Relaxation of the pelvic floor with a series of simple *blow when you go* exercises progressed Rita to where she could gently contract the pelvic floor once it had relaxed. With gradual progression of contraction followed by a controlled exhale, the tension in the pelvic floor dropped. Rita was then able to sit on a soft medicine ball without pain and a gradual progression of contractions gained Rita pelvic floor muscle support without pain.

Now that Rita was sensing less pain, she was able to more strongly contract the pelvic floor muscles. She noted particular ease in standing with the legs abducted (apart). Despite it normally being more difficult to overcome the disadvantageous lengthening of the muscle fibers, why did Rita find the abducted position more comfortable and thus easier to contract? Because the residual guarding likely positioned her muscle fibers with too much overlap for comfort. Think back to the length-tension curve whereby too much overlap of the pelvic floor muscles was also disadvantageous, likely due to pain. (See previous Figure 7a.) This pain seemed to have *masked* Rita's actual strength. Reduced pain with contraction appeared to make contracting the pelvic floor a more welcoming exercise. Eventually the contraction allowed for a lag time (discussed earlier in this section) when the muscles would somewhat relax before resuming a tense, guarded state. At this time, Rita would gently blow through pursed lips for relaxation. Strengthening occurred more rapidly once the initial pain barrier was removed. Increased voluntary control over the pelvic floor muscles improved with voluntary contraction and relaxation. Improved control allowed the muscles to have a normalized resting tone ready to contract against incontinence, and readily released for daily function without pain. (See Figure 31.)

Figure 31. An example of a re-evaluation of a patient having progressed with pelvic floor muscle tension release.

Diagnoses: Pelvic floor muscle spasms and weakness

Upon re-evaluation, the following were noted:
1. Patient is now strong enough to hold the pelvic floor in standing with hips abducted! She is able to do this in isolation of abdominals and gluteals for 5 seconds at a time, for intervals of 5 repetitions.
2. In being able to contract with hips abducted, patient is able to hold with significantly less pain in the pelvic cavity. This is likely due to a lesser amount of tension in the pelvic floor.
3. It is generally more difficult to hold a strong contraction when the hips are abducted due to disadvantageous lengthening. However, the patient appears to have the strength to contract. The pain associated with muscle tension appeared to hinder the contraction.
4. In releasing the muscle tension, strengthening will likely build for further pelvic floor control.
5. The ability to progressively contract and relax will also likely provide a normalized resting tone, furthering pain release.

Plan/Goals:
1. Independent with home exercise program-met.
2. Isolation of pelvic floor muscle contraction-met.
3. Full void and pelvic floor relaxation.
4. Resolution of pain with contraction in all positions.
5. Resolution of incontinence.

◆ ◆ ◆

Pelvic floor contraction may initially exacerbate the painful tension plaguing the pelvic floor, but that contraction is usually needed to eventually overcome it. Learning to at least partially relax the muscles first can ease the contraction. That contraction can then feed into the contract-relax cycle to eventually spiral down the pain. Rehabilitating the painful tension may initially feel like trudging uphill, in the sand, at a high altitude. But, once the initial relaxation and contraction are achieved, gaining further control can become easier and easier. Initial relaxation and contraction of the pelvic floor muscles are the rehabilitative pinnacles, and further pelvic floor control gaining momentum through successive treatments.

Chloe presented with right sacral outflare, right ilial elevation (malalignments of the sacrum and pelvis) and horrific pain throughout the pelvic region. She noted shooting pain across the inferior gluteals, (buttocks), down her right lower extremity, and into her foot. The pain into her lower extremity appeared to be a combination of sciatica (nerve pain stemming from the low back and sacrum) and soft tissue tension referral. Pain referral is the phenomenon whereby pain is felt in one region but stems from another. Chloe also noted pain along the sacroiliac joint, where the sacrum abuts the pelvis. Pain in the sacroiliac joint was resolved by correcting the outflare and the elevation (asymmetries). The pain that shot into the gluteals appeared to stem from compressive forces on the sacral nerves and on the pudendal nerve. Suspecting tension in the pelvic floor and its compressive forces on the nerves, the shooting pain was targeted with pelvic floor muscle tension release. A guided series of gentle contractions with full relaxation helped to relax the pelvic floor. Chloe also performed self-administered soft tissue mobilization to the pelvic floor muscles by sitting on the small medicine ball, which provided immediate relief. (Soft tissue mobilization is similar to massage, but very specific and directed at small regions of the body versus the body in its entirety.) Independent pelvic floor isolation and full relaxation exercises, and self-help asymmetry corrections complemented the treatments. It was important to remedy all sources of pain. Reducing the perineal muscles' compressive forces on the pudendal nerve branches and sacral roots, resolving the sacroiliac asymmetries, and gathering control of the pelvic floor muscles altogether relieved Chloe of the overwhelming pain of pelvic dysfunction.

A similar case to Chloe's was Jasmine's presentation of muscle guarding and pain, however Jasmine's guarding led to incomplete void with urinary urgency and frequency. Jasmine presented with right ilial (pelvic) elevation accompanied by quadratus lumborum (low back muscle) tension greater on the right than the left. Palpable tension in the pelvic floor muscles was significant enough to provoke sharp pain in the pelvic region. The right ilial (pelvic) elevation likely created a pulling sensation on the sacral nerve roots thereby tensing the pudendal nerve. The irritated pudendal nerve likely increased the pain and tension in Jasmine's pelvic floor muscles, leading to this probable series of events: Nerve irritation manifested as sharp pain in the pelvic region and tension in the muscles into which it fed. The muscle tension then compressed the nerve at the neuromuscular junction (where the nerve meets the muscle) creating more neural irritation in a vicious cycle. Such muscle tension in the pelvic floor not only constricted the urethra, it also sent a constant message to the brain's micturition center to counter the stretch reflex of the bladder's detrusor muscle. Following suit, the internal sphincter remained closed. Attempts to fully void were, therefore, likely not successful because the pelvic floor muscles could not fully relax.

As previously discussed in the section on incomplete void, a wavering series of contractions and relaxations of the pelvic floor can send flickering messages to the brain's micturition (voiding) center like a fluctuating supply of electricity inadequately powers a flickering light bulb. The pelvic floor's flickering contraction likely created a mixed message to Jasmine's micturition center, rendering a weak urine flow and a premature closing of the sphincter. The result was a frustratingly incomplete void. Without the ability to fully relax her pelvic floor to successfully void, Jasmine would feel the urge to urinate soon after leaving the restroom. Urgency surged from the confusion within her voiding circuit until the neural irritation subsided. Correction of the pelvic asymmetry eased the strain on the nerves. Improved neural integrity released the guarded musculature. Regaining control of the pelvic floor's contraction and relaxation disposed of Jasmine's micturition confusion, eased her voiding, and resolved her urgency.

Residual abdominal and pelvic pain may present after the sling surgery. Muscle guarding may result in difficulty releasing the pelvic floor contraction. (This muscle guarding in the pelvic floor is similar to that of the lower extremity muscles after a knee or hip surgery.) The release of the pelvic floor muscles is likely needed for full pain resolution as well as for complete voiding. Therefore, physical rehabilitation (physiotherapy) is often needed after sling surgery to maximize urinary control and remedy the residual pain, enhancing the overall success of the surgical procedure.

To exemplify, let me introduce Layla, an interesting case of significant pelvic floor muscle guarding after having had a sling surgery and a hysterectomy. Layla reported painful intercourse and difficulty voiding completely. She would attempt to fully empty her bladder, but then immediately sense a strong urge. The muscle guarding and readiness to clench likely stopped the stream too quickly, sending her rushing back to the restroom only minutes after having attempted to void.

The clenching that made voiding difficult also made for painful intercourse.

Layla stated her condition commenced 12 years prior to starting physical therapy, right after having a sling surgery and a hysterectomy. The muscles in a painfully guarded state included the pelvic floor and the iliacus, a hip flexor. Sitting on the small medicine ball placed between her anus and her vagina provided immediate relief, to the point where she promptly marched to the sporting goods store and bought her own! Tension in the iliacus (hip flexor) released with the first visit and further with the second. Teaching the patient to mobilize (or massage) and stretch the iliacus complimented the manual therapy I performed during treatment sessions. (See previous Figure 28.) With tension in the pelvic floor and iliacus (hip flexor) resolving, so was Layla's 12-year history of pain.

In short, as with the incomplete voiding scenario, pelvic pain can result from excessively contracted, guarded pelvic floor muscles. A full analysis of the patient can assist in finding sources of the pain. Treating the sources, such as pelvic asymmetry and neural entrapment, can keep noxious stimuli from feeding more tension into the pelvic floor. Sitting on the small medicine ball can act as a soft tissue mobilization or specific massage technique. Sitting on the large therapy ball and exhaling to release the contraction progressively can help to alleviate the pain. Controlled exhalation works in conjunction with the ball tricks to release tension and gradually resolve painful guarding of the pelvic floor.

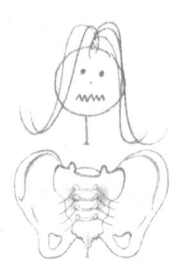

Dyspareunia

In my discussion of pelvic pain thus far, I have briefly touched upon the topic of painful intercourse. It is time to give that pain a name. *Dyspareunia* is the medical term for painful sexual intercourse. The pain with intercourse can stem from excess tension in the vaginal walls and pelvic floor muscles, and from reduced vaginal secretions. Furthermore, as one may hypothesize, persons with dyspareunia could also experience difficulty voiding due to the inability to fully relax the pelvic floor muscles and open the sphincters.

Muscle guarding, or excessive contraction, can stem from a number of sources of trauma and stress. Alterations in spinal alignment, as with scoliosis and spinal degeneration, can lead to painful compensatory pelvic shifts, which can also place the pelvic floor muscles en garde. Trauma, stress, and pelvic shifts not only can create weakness and pain in the pelvic region with outdoor activities, they can also wreak havoc in the bedroom!

Because Kegels can assist with training the pelvic floor muscles to contract *and relax*, I instruct my patients with dyspareunia to practice Kegels with an emphasis on the relaxation after the contractions, as with the *lava flow* exercise. Blowing through pursed lips, as when blowing to fully void, can often assist in achieving the muscle release patients need for pain resolution. Training patients to voluntarily contract and to fully relax the pelvic floor muscles can give them control over the pelvic floor's resting tone. Sitting on the small medicine ball can help reduce the tension in the pelvic floor muscles, as previously mentioned. (See previous Figure 31.) Lowering the tension or muscle tone to a comfortable level can ease sexual penetration. Control over the pelvic floor muscles can also improve sensation in this region. Improved sensation can lead to more vaginal secretions. Increasing vaginal secretions can assist in reducing friction with penetration. The lower the friction with penetration, the lower the pain with intercourse. Therefore, by reducing tension and pain, greater muscle release and greater secretions can lead to, well, greater sex!

For patients who do not see results with the Kegel contraction and relaxation, or for the patients that experience pain with a Kegel, electrical vaginal stimulation at a 200 Hz frequency can come to the rescue! The 200 Hz electrical stimulation can effectively assist in relaxing the pelvic floor muscles in patients with dyspareunia, just as it can in those experiencing incomplete void. The electrical stimulation alone can effectively ease the tension in the pelvic floor muscles, and, therefore, alleviate pain. If Kegeling is not painful, contracting then exercising the *blow when you go* technique to help the muscles relax, while receiving the stimulation, has reportedly allowed for even greater ease with relaxing. Either with or without the contract-relax exercises, adding 200 Hz electrical vaginal stimulation can result in less pelvic floor tension (detected with a biofeedback device) and reportedly ease pain with intercourse. When patients can Kegel without pain, I incorporate the contract-relax technique into their therapy. Training the muscles to relax after contracting is the ultimate goal, as it can improve a patient's control over her pelvic floor.

In using electrical vaginal stimulation to treat dyspareunia, I discovered that some patients had low levels of sensation in the vaginal region. Upon discovering the low level of sensation at 200 Hz, I tested the patients at the 50 and 12.5 Hz settings used by patients with stress urinary incontinence and urinary urgency respectively. Often, the patients with dyspareunia would only start to sense the stimulation at an average level *twice* that used by those who did not experience dyspareunia. Upon further inquisition, the patients with dyspareunia who had a low level of sensation would often divulge a lack of vaginal secretions with intercourse. Lack of adequate secretions likely compounded with the excess tension in the vaginal walls to worsen an already painful sexual experience. After an average of 4 treatments over the course of 2 weeks, sensation reportedly improved, and the patients would start to feel the electrical stimulation at lower and lower levels, eventually sensing the stimulation at the same average level as patients without dyspareunia. The sensation would vary from patient to patient, but overall, greater sensation was gained. In conjunction with increased sensation, the patients reported a greater amount of vaginal secretions during intercourse. Restored sensation with the help of Kegeling alone and Kegeling in conjunction with 200 Hz electrical vaginal stimulation, both appeared to correlate with increased vaginal secretions. Increases in vaginal secretions, along with tension reduction, can ease penetration and aid in having intercourse without pain.

I have treated several cases of dyspareunia that

presented in isolation of incomplete void. Such cases have often affiliated with emotional stress, relationship struggles, and/or sexual trauma. These cases highlight the importance of listening and allowing patients to divulge information at their own, comfortable pace. The physical aspects of dyspareunia can be treated with pelvic floor relaxation and voluntary contraction cues, and oftentimes with the assistance of 200 Hz electrical vaginal stimulation. These treatments can provide relief, however I have found that to truly resolve the condition, the negative emotional energy that resides in the pelvic region should be released. Oftentimes, this is not an easy task. Assisting patients can be as simple as listening. Other cases warrant the accompaniment of outside clinical assistance. Combining disciplines to treat the emotional anguish harnessed physically in the pelvic floor can successfully help patients overcome their trauma.

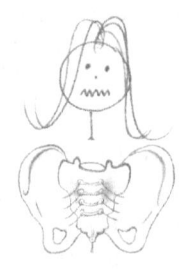

Dyspareunia, Cases in Point...

My next case will highlight the need to look outside the box for the source of a diagnosis...Amy presented with painful intercourse, incomplete void, and weak urine flow. She presented with significant tension in bilateral hip flexors, which reacted painfully to very gentle, grade 1 soft tissue mobilization of the iliacus (gentle massage of a hip flexor). What caused her condition? Gently extracting sensitive information, then inferring from her current conditions, I developed this hypothesis...

Amy simultaneously presented with nausea, inability to process spicy foods, and constant pain in her stomach and along the intestinal tract. Restricted hip flexors and tense erector spinae (low to mid back muscles) correlated with hyperlordosis (sway back). Amy's hyperlordosis commenced at the upper portion of the low back just beneath the ribs. (See Figure 32.) Such a sharp curve likely resulted in compression of the lower thoracic nerves, which feed into the stomach. Amy's *stomach point* just beneath the sternum presented with a painful tenderness and restriction as a result of digestive distress. Amy's tense and painful stomach point pulled her into a sidebend on the right. Her right hip flexor was more taut than the left, correlating with her side bent positioning. The greater tension in the right hip flexor created an anterior rotation of the right ilium. The right side of the pelvis was pulled more forward than the left. The altered length-tension relationship among her pelvic floor muscle fibers accompanying the pelvic asymmetry did not weaken the pelvic floor muscles enough to cause leaking, but it did appear to force the pelvic floor muscles into overexertion. Exertion of muscles fibers with disadvantageous configurations made countering incontinence and supporting the pelvic contents a difficult task. Such a strain to the pelvic floor likely prompted its muscle guarding.

Figure 32. An illustration of hyperlordosis stemming from the lower thoracic and upper lumbar regions with accompanied neural encroachment. The spinal segment encroaching upon exiting nerves from Figure 27 is also depicted.

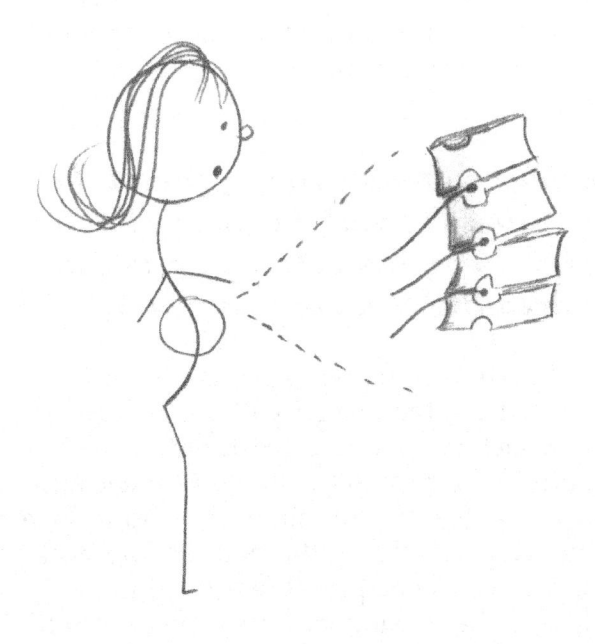

Applying gentle pressure to the stomach point can alleviate its tension and this tension release can trigger a domino effect of positive results. But, having someone else other than the patient touch this point can often create its own inherent guarding in anticipation of too great a force on a very delicate area. I had Amy self-administer the manual pressure, guiding her with gradual progression to release the tension in her stomach point. As the restrictions were released, Amy extended through the chest and mid back to lengthen the abdominal cavity. This lengthening stretched Amy's trunk eventually into an upright position. The tension release in the stomach point provided partial relief of her pain. Soft tissue mobilization (or massage) to the hip musculature and symmetrical alignment of the pelvis further eased Amy's pain and restored adequate pelvic floor muscle fiber length. Adequate muscle fiber length likely helped to resolve overexertion and strain. Eliminating the strain appeared to cease the pelvic floor muscle guarding, and adequate recovery was had.

"I can't believe someone finally found the source of my stomach pain! I came to therapy for pelvic pain. Now, my pelvic pain is gone, and so is that dreadful tension in my stomach!"

To remedy the digestive distress causing Amy's stomach point to constrict, the integrity of the nerves innervating her stomach needed to be restored. Application of manual therapy to the lower thoracic and upper lumbar paraspinals (muscles along the mid to lower spine) reduced the tension holding the swayed low back in hyperlordosis. The newly acquired neutral spine consequently released the tension irritating the nerves that innervated her stomach. Releasing the tension that compressed the lower thoracic nerves resolved the source of Amy's digestive distress. Resolving the digestive distress resolved the tension harnessed in her stomach point, which, in turn, allowed Amy to assume erect posture. Amy's erect posture complemented the manual therapy (massage) applied to the low back and hip flexor muscles. Releasing tension in the low back and hip flexor muscles allowed the pelvis to realign. Realigning the ilia (sides of pelvis) improved the length-tension relationship among the pelvic floor's muscle fibers allowing them to contract without overstraining. Alleviating the pelvic floor's strain and training the pelvic floor to contract and relax without guarding finally restored normal voiding and resolved Amy's dyspareunia. Amy's overall presentation clearly required a holistic healing approach, as each of her conditions intertwined with the others creating a snowball effect …Hence my emphasis on looking beyond the pelvic floor to treat the pelvic floor in full capacity!

On her last day of therapy, Amy excitedly remarked, "I can't believe someone finally found the source of my stomach pain! I came to therapy because of my pelvic pain. Now, my pelvic pain is gone, and so is that dreadful tension in my stomach!" Amy, like other patients, was thrilled to live life pain free. As each condition was resolved, Amy's relief built like a snowball bowling down a mountain. Her overall pain dropped to nothing. Peeling back the layers of ailments and finding their sources were necessary in order to truly rehabilitate Amy's dyspareunia. Resolving those ailments along the way was the proverbial icing.

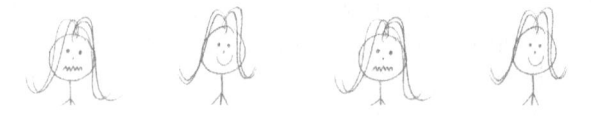

Dyspareunia with Pain in Flux

Some patients with dyspareunia report wavering levels of pain, ranging from unbearable to barely existent. These cases may not involve any apparent physical trauma, however, an underlying tension may develop insidiously, gradually worsen, then subside. Wavering levels of mental or emotional stress may correlate with fluctuating degrees of dyspareunia, which seems to have been the case for several of my patients. Stress levels may not elevate enough to throw the patients into autonomic survival mode, but they can hit a high enough point to cause the pelvic floor muscles to clench in a guarded state. The resulting sustained muscle tension disrupts full urine flow and makes intercourse painfully unpleasant.

Patients with fluctuating dyspareunia may be able to isolate and fully relax the pelvic floor, but the length of time the patients can sustain relaxation may be the problem. Shayla was able to fully relax, but only for a short period of time. She found herself clenching the pelvic floor muscles within 2 seconds of relaxation. Electrical vaginal stimulation set at 200Hz catalyzed Shayla's ability to relax the pelvic floor for longer and longer periods, eventually allowing for pain free intercourse. Shayla lived a life full of stress, knowing that her husband was on the battlefield at any given time of day or night. Even when her husband was home, the stress of knowing that he would once again leave for combat attacked her pelvic floor muscles. She had not been able to manage her muscle gripping stress, but when her husband was home from combat, she wanted to be able to enjoy his company in *every* way! The 200 Hz electrical vaginal stimulation was her savior in the intercourse department. We discussed ways for her to de-stress, but had not come to a conclusion before she and her husband relocated to a new duty station. She practiced Kegels with full relaxation to eventually regain control over her pelvic floor muscles even in stressful situations. But, because the stimulation was the magic element that relieved the tension in a pinch (literally and figuratively), she bought a stimulator to use independently. The stimulators are quite expensive, but she emphatically stated that having a means to alleviate the pelvic floor muscle tension was worth every penny!

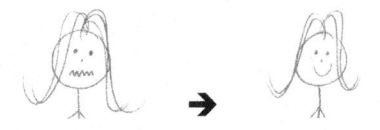

A Sneak Attack on Dyspareunia

Patients with dyspareunia have unexpectedly stumbled upon treatment because they sought care for another ailment. These patients were often unaware that dyspareunia could resolve with physical therapy, so they did not bother to mention their symptoms. However, hints that patients have dyspareunia can creep up on clinicians as patients treated for cervical (neck) or shoulder conditions gradually divulge information about themselves. These hints can lead to successful, and surprising, rehabilitation…

Lucy was being treated for cervical pain, but in

discussing her other ailments she disclosed symptoms that spelled dyspareunia. I eased into a conversation about how common dyspareunia was and how therapy can resolve pain with intercourse. Furthering this discussion, she reported a loss of libido when she stopped taking oral contraceptives. While taking the oral contraceptives, the ingested hormones may have induced a libido as such hormones can mimic being pregnant. Upon discontinuing the oral contraceptives, she also reportedly stopped producing vaginal secretions. I speculate that having taken an outside source of hormones may have altered Lucy's natural regulation of excretion, similar to the way that taking pain medications can disrupt the body's natural production of pain relievers. Without vaginal secretions, intercourse became painfully unbearable. Painful intercourse would rightfully dissuade any sexual desire…Hence the dwindling of Lucy's libido. But, the loss of vaginal secretions was not the only cause of her dyspareunia. A number of factors were revealed as her story unfolded.

    Lucy's pelvic floor muscles could relax enough to allow urine to flow through and exit the urethra, but would not relax during intercourse as they would when she took the oral contraceptives. Losing the production of vaginal secretions made penetration painful. The anticipation of pain could have added to the tension in the pelvic floor making relaxation with penetration impossible. Lucy's pelvic floor muscles would relax to allow partial penetration, but clench abruptly when she sensed pain along the vaginal walls. It appeared as though Lucy's pain with full penetration enhanced the pelvic floor's muscle guarding and further hindered secretions that would, in a situation devoid of pain, arrive with positive stimulation. Alas, a downward spiral of pain and guarding with diminished secretions ensued...Goodbye libido, hello dyspareunia!

Lucy, like many a patient with dyspareunia, thought she was able to relax the pelvic floor because she did not have trouble voiding. But, a 10-year history of right ilial elevation and anterior rotation (pelvic malalignments) seemed to have contributed to a tension in her pelvic floor that was difficult to *fully* release. The strain of having to provide organ support and continence with overly lengthened muscle fibers likely irritated the pelvic floor muscles enough to cause them to partially guard. The guarding likely hindered full relaxation during intercourse. This pent up tension plus the additional guarding caused by painful penetration on top of a loss of vaginal secretions likely combined to make intercourse for Lucy very painful.

Treatment for Lucy's dyspareunia began with aligning the pelvis to alleviate the pelvic floor strain, and exercising to gain better control over the pelvic floor muscles. To correct the obliquities, the right side of the low back and the right hip flexor muscles were treated with soft tissue mobilization (specific massage) and stretches. (See previous Figures 16a, 16b, and 28.) To gain better control over the pelvic floor, Lucy repeatedly performed a Kegel then concentrated on relaxing her pelvic floor muscles with the *lava flow* exercise while sitting on a large therapy ball. As Lucy sat on the ball, she relaxed in successive waves, and realized that she had *not* been fully relaxing. By contracting first, then relaxing, she was able to feel the therapy ball's tactile pressure in a descending and outward moving pattern, signaling the much needed, full relaxation of the pelvic floor.

To further assist with relaxation, Lucy utilized 200 Hz electrical vaginal stimulation. The stimulation not only relaxed the pelvic floor to help Lucy overcome the painful tension, it also reportedly restored Lucy's tactile sensation in a positive way. Heightened sensation drew even greater vaginal secretions. Greater vaginal secretions further eased penetration, reducing chances of pain, and therefore reducing chances of guarding. The tension release and the promotion of vaginal secretions, achieved with the 200 Hz electrical vaginal stimulation, ultimately assisted in reducing Lucy's pain.

Strain Release → Tension Release → Pain Relief →

Secretion Release → Greater Tension Release →

Greater Pain Relief →

Resolution of Dyspareunia ☑

Lucy's previous idea of a fully relaxed pelvic floor paled in comparison to what she could achieve after having physical therapy. Successive treatments to stabilize pelvic symmetry resolved the strain that the malalignments had placed on the pelvic floor muscle fibers. Resolving the strain on her pelvic floor muscles potentiated full relaxation. Having a greater potential to fully relax, the pelvic floor could release with the help of the lava flow exercises and the 200 Hz electrical stimulation. Relaxing the pelvic floor allowed for a greater opening of the perineal orifices. Lucy's anxiety of the possibility of pain with intercourse diminished and the anxiety's inherent guarding disappeared. Penetration provided a positive response (versus a clenching due to pain) and electrical stimulation helped to promote vaginal secretions. Greater ease in opening the vaginal walls and greater flow of vaginal secretions allowed for painless intercourse, and Lucy's libido was revived! (Oh! And as for her neck pain, therapy resolved that as well.)

Dyspareunia can stem from a myriad of impairments which cause pent up tension in the pelvic floor. Dissecting each cause and treating of each and every one of the impairments can lead to full resolution. One factor can lead to another, like tension leading to pain, pain leading to secretion cessation, secretion cessation leading to more pain. But, just as readily as the dominoes fall, they can be picked back up. Resolving the tension helps resolve the pain. And without the anxiety of the pain, secretions rebound. Yes, physical therapy with a very holistic approach can work wonders in resolving dyspareunia! But, Lucy's case, like so many cases of dyspareunia, likely would have gone untreated had she not been in therapy for another diagnosis. She had no idea that physical therapy could treat dyspareunia. This is one of the reasons why I wrote this book! To get the word out that there is hope in returning to pleasurable intercourse!

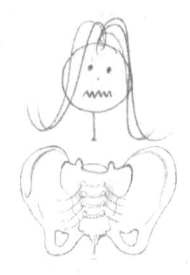

A Handful of Conditions Associated with Pelvic Pain:

Endometriosis and Interstitial Cystitis, Tumors, Calcified Masses, and Uterine Fibroids

Interstitial cystitis and endometriosis are common culprits of pelvic pain. Both involve pain and inflammation of pelvic organs, and potentiate scar tissue development.[44,45]

Interstitial cystitis is an inflammation of the bladder. Bloating and cramping are common accompaniments, resembling severe premenstrual symptoms. A body's inflammatory response in cases of interstitial cystitis may subside if there is more support for the bladder with sound pelvic floor musculature. The pelvic floor supports the bladder, and thus keeps the bladder positionally intact. Such support protects against a jolting or a falling sensation of the bladder that could trigger an inflammatory response.[44,45]

Endometriosis is a condition whose cause is elusive and whose treatments follow suit. With the menstrual cycle, the uterus is lined with endometrial tissue to ready the implantation of the zygote. Should impregnation not occur, the endometrial lining is normally shed with menstruation. Should the lining fail to shed, endometriosis may unfortunately develop. In some cases, the endometrial cells may travel to the Fallopian tubes, the ovaries, the cervix, and to other tissues outside of the boundaries of the uterus. This build up of excess tissue can quite possibly create pain, as the tissue may tug on the organs to which it is attached.[44,45]

According to Dr. David Redwine, a specialist in laproscopic excision of endometriosis, endometriosis may stem from a different cause: A misplacement of endometrial cells throughout a female's development. Some cells may land appropriately as endometrial lining, but others may land inappropriately in other regions of the body such as in the intestinal tract, on the ovaries, or in the Fallopian tubes.[46]

As I will elaborate later with case scenarios, I am a firm believer in the latter endometriosis scenario. Sensing a palpable difference in muscle tissue anywhere from the mid back to the hip muscles, I feel that the misplaced cells go even beyond the pelvic cavity.

Uterine fibroids are abnormally excessive growths of the uterine tissues. These growths are benign tumors but can grow to incredible measures.[47] The largest I have personally seen was 7 inches in diameter! Fibroids may sit in the walls of the uterus pressing against the inner and outer layers. Such pressure can lead to painful disruption of tissue spaces leading to pain not only in the uterus, but also in the low back and pelvic musculature.[46]

Malignant tumors may present throughout the abdominal cavity and its organs, as can cysts and calcified masses. The presence of tumors, cysts, and calcified masses can apply pressure on the contents of the abdominal and pelvic cavities as the fibroids can to the uterus. Furthermore, the surfaces of such can be abrasive, feeling like crusty, rusted steel wool scratching and tearing at muscles, ligaments, tendons, and organs as the weight of the abdominal cavity's contents is carried.

This weight of the abdominal cavity's contents can pull on the scar tissue and endometrial tissue, and tug on the fibroids, tumors, cysts, and calcified masses, provoking pain. A painful tearing sensation can arise, as can an inflammatory response. This inflammation can lead to more pressure, more pain, and more pulling, all of which can add to the pain of having a mass intrude upon an organs' personal space. When daily activities jolt and pull on the existing scar tissue, the tissue can tear and more scar tissue can build to remediate.

The pain response I have seen appears to be threefold. The first pain response seems to be directly caused by the extraneous and/or inflamed tissues pressing against abdominal contents and tugging at host tissues in which they are embedded. The second appears to arise from the body's inflammatory response in the surrounding muscles, tendons, and ligaments, and in the abnormality's host tissues. Guarding in the pelvic cavity can ensue just like the ankle muscles can acquire tension in order to support a sprained ligament. The third seems to emerge from a forwardly flexed (hunched) posture generated in response to such pain, which, in turn, can cause more pain.

When in pain, the natural response is to hunch forward, as with a stomachache or a swift kick to the groin. Imagine that pain 10 fold, constantly. Instead of standing upright and allowing the scratchy calcified masses to tear at the tissues in which they are embedded, patients tend to remain hunched, minimizing any movement in the abdomen. This posture can eventually lead to the tightening and straining of the muscles that are most likely already guarded and restricted due to the inflammatory response.

With a forwardly flexed, hunched posture, the iliopsoas muscles (hip flexors), abdominals, and pectorals (chest muscles) can tighten due to being in a shortened position. Strained hip extensors and extensors of the lumbar and thoracic regions (low back and mid back) can result from working in a disadvantageously lengthened position in attempts to hold the trunk as upright as the culprits of pain allow. The forwardly flexed lumbar (low back) position sets the stage for a disc bulge or herniation and the accompanying nerve irritation. The flexed trunk positioning can also lead to cervical pain due to a compensatory forward head position. While hunched in a flexed position, excessive cervical (neck) extension or jutting is usually needed for the patients to see ahead of them. Otherwise, they would be forced to look at the ground. What problems can a forward head create? Jutting the head forward can lead to joint and disc degeneration in the cervical and upper thoracic spines (neck and upper back) and degeneration's associated neural irritation. Alas, the saga of abnormal and excess pelvic tissues unfolds, potentiating a tangling web of secondary and tertiary traumas screaming for the help of rehabilitation.

With the multiple sources of pain, pelvic disorders should not be addressed by staring narrowly at the pelvic floor. Keeping the extraneous motion of the masses and tearing of the embedded tissues to a minimum is certainly of utmost importance, and a strong pelvic floor can act as a base, or scaffolding, if you will, to hold the contents in an upright position. Holding the organs in place as such can unweight the scar tissue surrounding the organs. This unweighting can reduce the pulling sensation on the existing scar tissue, reduce pain, reduce the formation of future scar tissue, and thusly reduce the cyclical inflammatory responses. However, addressing the subsequently acquired conditions and teaching sound body mechanics to minimize exacerbations of secondary and tertiary pain are also significant! Hence the importance of astute, open-minded, holistic physical (physio-) therapy in the realm of pelvic pain rehabilitation.

"Nothing stopped the pain like physical therapy."

Several of my patients with pelvic pain conditions have reported a lack of success with prescribed medications including hormone treatments. Many clinicians treat endometriosis with anti-inflammatories, oral contraceptives, and medications that stop estrogen production so as to mimic menopause. These oral contraceptives and gonadotropin agonists aim to reduce the addition of further endometrial tissue in outlying regions such as the ovaries and colon, external to the uterus.[48] However, even if further layering of endometrial tissue is halted, the pain associated with the previous layering of tissue is still alive. Time and again my patients have told me, "Nothing stopped the pain like physical [physio-] therapy".

Some of the pain associated with endometriosis has been reported in the pelvis and low back. This pain may stem straight from inflammatory fluid building up and stagnating in these regions, or from organs irritated by the layering of out-of-place endometrial tissue. A sense of guarding can erupt in the pelvic musculature, like the calf and shin muscles can guard after spraining an ankle. The muscles surrounding the pelvic cavity can resort to a protective mode, but that protective mode in itself can be painful.

The iliopsoas (hip flexor) is a usual suspect caught harnessing painful symptoms associated with pelvic cavity dysfunction. Two separate hip flexors, the iliacus and the psoas, merge to create the aptly named iliopsoas muscle. The iliopsoas crosses the hip region and attaches onto the femur of the lower extremity. All three hip flexor components, the iliacus, the psoas, and the iliopsoas, may develop painful tension in a guarded state. Such tension can add to the pain, and add to the possibility of developing lumbar hyperlordosis (sway back). (See previous Figure 27.) If both the right and the left sided iliopsoas muscles are restricted, they can together sway the lumbar spine. If one side is tighter than the other, asymmetry can occur across the pelvis. The tighter of the two can create a unilateral anterior ilial rotation (cause only one side of the pelvis to rotate). (See previous Figure 10a.) The symmetrical and the asymmetrical rotations of the pelvis can birth lumbar, thoracic, and sacral soft tissue tension and pain. Soft tissue mobilization (specific massage) and moist heat, followed by gentle, gradually progressive hip flexor stretches can alleviate hip flexor tension. Tension release can allow for ilial symmetry and a neutral spine, which define positions affording the least amount of strain in the surrounding tissues. Core conditioning can stabilize the resumed alignment, and the surrounding soft tissues can cease guarding. Retraining adequate control and establishing a normalized resting tone in the iliopsoas can come with controlled contraction and relaxation exercises. Controlled tone can help to minimize recurrence of excessive tension. With resolution of iliopsoas tension, one of the regulars on the pelvic pain scene is put to rest.

Other potential harnessers of tension in the realm of pelvic pain include the piriformis, tensor fascia latae, gemellus, gluteus medius, gluteus minimus, gluteus maximus, and obturator internus and externus all in the pelvic and hip regions, and the lumbar and thoracic paraspinals of the low and mid back. The tension harnessed within these muscles can run deep. Breaking barriers of the pain can require successive steps with gradual release of the outer layers before breaking up the tension in the inner layers. Too much force with soft tissue mobilization (massage) can set the muscles into a tailspin of regression as the pain can ignite the inflammation process and create even more tension. The mobilization (massage) of these muscles should be only as strong as the muscles allow and the patient deems comfortable. By palpating the muscles, the clinician can feel if the muscles give in or push away. Gentle, short-lived pressure applications can make way for longer holds gradually releasing the tension. Scar tissue that has grown between the muscle fibers out of stagnation can be gently broken. Gradual conditioning can train the muscle fibers to adequately contract once again and release to recover. Throughout this process, communication between the clinician and the patient is an absolute must. Sometimes muscle soreness develops after manual therapy or exercise. Latent effects of treatments and home exercises, such as delayed onset of muscle soreness, should be addressed to determine whether a "good" pain, as with muscle conditioning, was had, or a state of painful inflammation had set the muscles into a tizzy. Like other aspects of therapy, the patient and clinician should work as a team. Mobilization and conditioning of hip, pelvic, low back, and mid back musculature should be a team effort to most effectively release the tension of the pained muscles that strike with dysfunctions of the pelvic cavity.

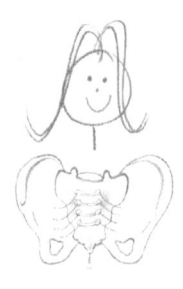

The Role of the Core in Fighting Pelvic Pain

The deep abdominal musculature, the transverse abdominis, is a star player in keeping the pelvis and spine in neutral positions. Without the inner abdominal strength to hold the lumbar spine in neutral, the pelvis can tilt anteriorly. Anterior pulling can tug at the walls of the abdomen, and contribute to the aforementioned pain cycle.

Furthermore, without transverse abdominis contraction the pelvic floor may have to work doubly hard as the foundation of core stability. Overworking the pelvic floor can lead to inflammation, guarding, and inadequate control over contraction and relaxation. The pelvic floor can fatigue when recovery time is lost and contraction is on overdrive. Without the ability to relax, urine can be retained, intercourse can be painful, and the pelvic floor itself can perpetuate an overuse injury! Therefore, if scar tissue has developed in the abdominal cavity as with interstitial cystitis, endometriosis, or with surgeries and fibroids, it behooves a patient with pelvic pain to gain control over the pelvic floor *and* the transverse abdominis. Gaining control in the full core can supply greater underlying and overlying support to the pelvis's organs by holding the spine and pelvis in place. Full core control can minimize imbalanced muscle recruitment and guarded muscle tension, and can minimize the painful consequences of pelvic malalignment.

In training the contraction of the full core, let me re-emphasize the importance of first mastering an isolated Kegel. The pelvis's scaffolding should be strongly in place before adding abdominal pressure. Otherwise, the abdominal pressure could strike an episode of incontinence. With the Kegel established, the full core can be introduced, but in doing so I advise contracting the pelvic floor first then adding the transverse abdominis. The transverse abdominis is targeted by gently pulling the navel to the spine. Breathing through the diaphragm while contracting the pelvic floor and transverse abdominis completes the core contraction for full trunk support. For a patient that also has incontinence, I recommend continuing a series of isolated Kegel contractions separate from a series of full core exercises. This is another instance whereby I have the patient think of herself as 2 separate patients so as to not confuse continence control with incorporation of any muscles other than the pelvic floor. This can be a tricky situation because the pelvic floor may be overworked as the sole provider of core support if the inner abdominals are not in check. But, the separation of Kegeling for continence and Kegeling for core support can address the pelvic floor's dual function and eventually result in full rehabilitation of both.

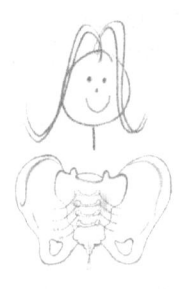

Nutrition, a Pelvic Pain Fighter

As a professional athlete, I have done my fair share of research on dietary needs for performance and recovery, and as a clinician, I have shared that knowledge with patients to speed their recovery from bouts of pelvic pain. I was dissatisfied with searches in medical publications for nutritional advice, so I looked to those that create the nutrition for a living. In my opinion, the entities with the biggest interests in recovery and performance nutrition research are the companies that are built on those very products. I have used my own personal experiences with nutrition to make recommendations with the caveat that each individual person and condition can respond uniquely to different nutrients. Drawing from a long history of athletic performance and digging through articles on athletes' successful nutrition, I have accumulated helpful hints to minimize cramping and painful bloating, as well as tips to improve the recovery rates of strained tissues. Patients want to overcome injured, inflamed tissues, just as athletes want recover from the microtears and inflammation associated with workouts and races. Nutrition can assist in alleviating the pain associated with pelvic inflammation and muscle tension as it can speed the recovery from an arduous day of athletics on the trail, on the track, on the road, and on the water. Educating patients about the nutrition that has helped me train for, win, and recover from grueling races has complemented the hands-on and exercise aspects of rehabilitation, holistically propelling patients toward recovery.

If proper electrolytes can curb muscle cramping and fluid retention in athletes, why not recommend electrolytes to patients suffering from cramps and fluid retention?

Well, I have recommended such electrolytes to my patients, and my patients have had great success following my recommendations. Fluid retention and cramping can be evils for those in athletic competition as well as for those in need of pelvic pain rehabilitation, and doubly so for those competing while needing rehabilitation! For athletes, fluid retention and cramps can be race stopping, winning streak ending, heartbreaking evils. Those very evils sparked my initial research. Similarly, fluid retention and cramping may be gut-wrenching, literally and figuratively, for a patient with pelvic inflammation. A proper electrolyte balance is necessary for athletic success, and for recovery from daily activities while battling pelvic pain. Essential fluid transport, tissue function, and tissue recovery depend on electrolyte balance. This balance helps to promote quality motor function and tissue recovery for athletes fighting to win, as it does for patients fighting to overcome pelvic pain.

Nutrition's Fight Against Pelvic Pain in a Bit More Detail

To recover from the excess tension associating with pelvic pain, the pelvic, hip, and back muscles need fuel and hydration. Protein helps rebuild tissue. Proper hydration helps flush out metabolites built up in the cells after cellular digestion and energy production. Fluid retained between the muscle tissue and the skin suggests an imbalanced system that can be restored to normalcy with the assistance of electrolytes. Fruits and vegetables with adequate electrolytes, such as potassium, and vitamins, such as vitamin C are key players in reducing inflammation and rebuilding broken down tissue.[49,50] Free radicals accumulate with inflammation and break down tissues. Vitamin C in oranges and pears can act as an antioxidant, which strips the free radicals of their destructive power, helping to get the tissues on the road to recovery. Bananas, with their potassium, can help keep water in the muscle tissues minimizing cramps and maximizing strength output. Without potassium, the water needed for muscle function can seep between the muscles and the skin, which can lead to bloating.[49,50] Cucumbers and lemons can further flush fluids that accumulate with inflammation. These foods work well to minimize cramping and/or fluid retention accompanying inflammation,[51] likely due to their constituent water molecules and electrolytes. Minimizing cramping and fluid retention with nutrition can help fight pain and reduce pressure on strained tissues. Reducing the pain and the strain helps keep inflammation at bay. By helping to suppress inflammation and restore tissue health, proper nutrition can accelerate patients' recovery from dreadful episodes of pelvic pain.

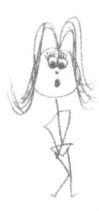

Nutrients that Flush Retained Fluid May Increase Bladder Irritation...

What is a Woman To Do?

Renee presented with endometriosis and interstitial cystitis with their accompanied painful fluid retention. Bloating increased pain and pressure on an already irritated bladder. This painful pressure likely contributed to her urinary frequency of once per hour in the daytime and four times per night. Renee also presented with incomplete void. Muscle tension in a guarded pelvic floor was once again the likely cause of urinary retention. Incomplete voids kept Renee in *'go mode'* sending her back to the restroom within 20 minutes of having urinated. To add insult to injury, chemical irritants were found to cause Renee's bladder to contract prematurely, increasing untimely urges and promoting urinary frequency.

Renee noted increased severity of bladder pain with particular foods. It just so happened that all of the foods Renee mentioned were on the *'Unhappy Bladder'* list including oranges, tomatoes, and lemons. (See previous Figure 22.) She did note, however, that she tolerated water infused with citrus fruits such as oranges and lemons. The infusion was a perfect example of what I call *putting out the fire*. Foods listed as bladder irritants can often be consumed with less or no irritation to the bladder if accompanied by water. As previously mentioned, citrus fruits can assist in reducing water retained between the muscles and the skin, as do cucumbers and bananas.[51] Consuming citrus infused water granted Renee vitamin and antioxidant nourishment and assistance in reducing fluid retention, without citrus-induced premature contraction of the bladder's detrusor muscle and without bladder pain.

    In conjunction with minimizing irritant-induced bladder contraction, Renee's urinary frequency improved with *lava flow* exercises, with the *'blow when you go'* technique, with a timed voiding schedule with progressively greater periods between voids, and with Kegeling repeatedly for 2 seconds or less. The *lava flow* exercises and the *'blow when you go'* technique improved upon her complete voids. The timed voiding schedule minimized the untimely contractions of her bladder and gave Renee control over her urination schedule. The Kegels helped to strongly message Renee's micturition center to inhibit premature bladder contraction and internal sphincter opening. With greater control over her bladder, Renee was able to consume citrus fruits by better countering the detrusor's citrus-induced contractions. Drinking water with these fruits was still recommended, though, in order to minimize a recurrence of chemical irritation. Reducing the chance of chemical irritation aimed to reduce overall pain and bladder irritation in the event of an exacerbation of pain and inflammation with interstitial cystitis.

    The *lava flow, 'blow when you go',* and Kegel exercises also better conditioned Renee's pelvic floor muscles allowing them to create a stronger scaffold to help hold her bladder in place. Long 10-second Kegels followed by *lava flow* exercises improved Renee's control over her pelvic floor muscles, giving the muscles a greater ability to contract and to recover from use. Improved ability to contract and recover improved the pelvic floor's readiness to support the bladder against jolts of intra-abdominal pressure. Greater support to the bladder helped reduce the irritating affect of jolting that can add to the inflammation associated with interstitial cystitis.

Turmeric: A Natural Anti-Inflammatory

Can Turmeric Impede Estrogen's Promotion of Endometriosis?

Quite possibly. Turmeric is widely known as a natural anti-inflammatory. There is speculation that turmeric may act as a natural contraceptive by keeping the uterus from preparing for implantation of the fertilized egg, essentially countering the estrogen's effects on increasing endometrial cells lining the uterus. Furthermore, there is speculation that turmeric counters the estrogen-induced building of the endometrial cells in the cervix. It appears as though Indian medicine and Chinese medicine have been embracing turmeric for years to minimize fibroids and endometriosis, but I have not yet found Western literature to support such. With anti-inflammatory and anti-coagulant properties, turmeric may be a pain relieving spice and an ingredient in improving upon inflammation and endometriosis.[52]

Several patients have stated that they have been turned away from turmeric because it disrupts their synthetic oral contraceptive's effectiveness, particularly affecting estrogen levels. If higher estrogen levels promote endometriosis, then why not use the turmeric instead of contraceptive pills? The pills often also contain progesterone, which keeps the uterus lined in preparation for pregnancy. In treating endometriosis, we are trying to rid the uterus of the excess lining. Therefore, why not try turmeric, which may minimize the accumulation of the lining, instead of a pill that, aside from having estrogen, also has progesterone, which may prolong it?

The contraceptive pills do attempt to inhibit ovulation, and ovulation can be very painful in patients with endometriosis. Perhaps the increase in levels of luteizing hormone, which promotes ovulation, is inhibited when taking Western oral contraceptives.[53] If turmeric disrupts the effect of the pills, ovulation may be disinhibited. Furthermore, I understand that some contraceptives work to line the cervix in order to promote a physical barrier to the swimming sperm. The turmeric may reduce this lining. However, the turmeric also reduces the lining of the uterus, and without that lining the zygote cannot attach. There are many substances that interfere with synthetic contraceptives, such as antibiotics. But, turmeric seems to get the bad rap. Being skeptical of turmeric's so called rap sheet, I think it is worth giving turmeric a shot at helping to minimize endometriotic pain.

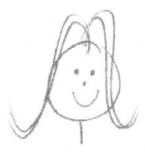

The Power of the Healing Touch: Diagnostic and Therapeutic

In some patients with pelvic pain stemming from endometriosis, fibroids, and interstitial cystitits, I have seen and felt excess tension in the lower thoracic and upper lumbar region, namely the thoraco-lumbar junction where the low back's concavity and the mid back's convexity meet. One patient carried her children on the right ilium or side of pelvis. Another habitually stood with the right side of her pelvis elevated in a "hip-hiked" position. Is the excess tension in these patients' muscles due to endometriosis, or bad posture, or a combination of both? I have treated several patients presenting with such posture who did not also have endometriosis. It appeared as though the patients without endometriosis healed more quickly from the elevated positioning. It is possible that more scar tissue accumulates in those with endometriosis. But is the excess tension in the back and low back muscles due to scar tissue or actual endometriotic tissue embedded in these muscles? I side with the latter.

Having palpated muscles on a plethora of patients, I have noticed a stark difference in the texture among those with and those without endometriosis. Four cases of endometriosis presented similarly with a distinct texture noted in the lower thoracic paraspinal muscles (muscles along the mid back), in the iliopsoas (hip flexor), and particularly in the iliacus (hip flexor). This textured tension appeared to wax and wane, similar to an endometriotic pattern. A visual of endometriotic tissue is similar to that of a group of adipose (fat) cells. The endometriotic cells, like adipose, may always be present, but may not always be full. The fullness of the endometriotic tissue may result from inflammation.[54] Increases in the muscles' tension may be due to endometriotic flares, with cyclical inflammation in the presence of estrogen. Three of the 4 patients with this presentation had undergone excision of the endometriotic tissue in the uterus. The fourth had not had the surgery as of yet. It had not been determined whether residual endometriotic cells had embedded in the muscle tissue or inflammatory scar tissue had developed. But, in all of these cases, the mid back, low back, and hip flexor muscles presented with the same texture. This *endometriotic texture* did not necessarily correlate with the patients' activity, it correlated with having endometriosis, even if excision surgery to remove endometriotic tissue from the uterus was had. I firmly believe the tissue I sensed was endometriotic. This speculation would tie in nicely with Dr. Redwine's theory that misplaced cells during development can lead to endometriosis.[46] Even after excision surgery removes the endometriotic tissue elsewhere, I believe endometriosis can remain embedded in the muscle tissue, which would explain the distinct texture.

As compared to other tissue textures, the *endometriotic texture* is tougher, like that of a low-grade steak, and more sinewy if you will. As a pre-teen, I volunteered to work the snack shack at my younger brother's little league games. The old, nearly encrusted bubbles of oil appearing after an evening of deep-frying French fries come to mind when I palpate the aforementioned muscles. These muscles feel like coarse fibers filled with pockets of old, used vegetable oil that had been sitting in a deep fryer. The tough, sinewy, bubble-encrusted texture is quite distinct to the muscles in my patients with endometriosis, whether they had excision surgery or not.

For the muscles sporting the *endometriotic texture*, soft tissue mobilization (massage) can make them less sinewy, less bubbly, less restricted, and less painful. Once the mobility is restored, a gradual strengthening regime can begin to condition the muscles. Starting the conditioning in a gravity-assisted position can provide for exercise without overexertion. Such a position is supine. Lying on her back, the patient can raise her arms one at time for counterforce exertion of the paraspinals (muscles along the spine). Hip extension with bridges may help the lower thoracic and lumbar (mid and low back) muscles to contract and relax for conditioning purposes. Complementing the soft tissue mobilization (massage), conditioning can teach these muscles to contract and relax, releasing them from their habitually guarded and tense state.

To minimize inflammation, strengthening and stretching can help to keep the underlying baseline of muscle tension at bay. To maximize the effects and longevity of the mobility and tension release obtained with hands-on therapy to the hip flexors and spinal muscles, stretching those muscles is recommended as part of the home exercise program. (See previous Figure 28 and see Figure 33.) The inflammation may also be treated with natural anti-inflammatories such as turmeric. Together manual soft tissue mobilization, postural correction, muscle conditioning, and natural anti-inflammatories can help keep the potential endometriotic cells 'deflated'. The sinewy, bubbly sensation can disappear and reappear as the endometriosis can wax and wane. However, with repeated physical therapy sessions addressing the sinewy muscles, I have noticed a pattern of increased longevity without the *endometriotic texture* and a return of the smoother texture mimicking muscles without endometriosis.

Figure 33. An illustration depicting stretches of the thoracic paraspinals (mid back muscles).

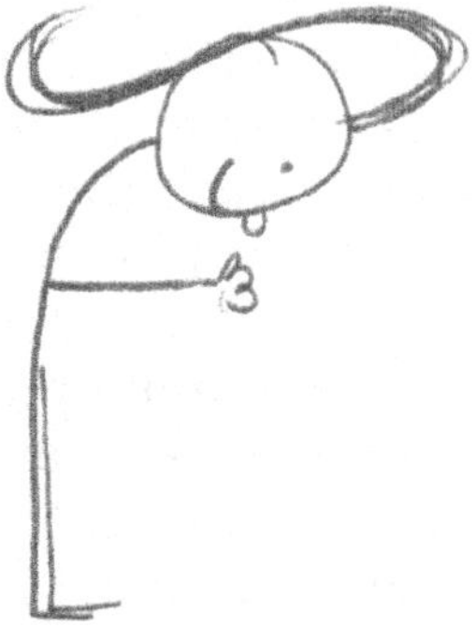

There seems to be a connection between tension in the hip flexor muscles and inflammation in the abdomen. The inflammation I am referring to is a distinct protrusion of the lower abdominal region that disappears almost immediately with release of the iliacus and iliopsoas muscles (hip flexors). The hypertensive muscles likely compress lymphatic ducts, which are vessels that help drain fluid from tissues. The iliacus joins the psoas to form the iliopsoas muscle, which attaches onto the femur (thigh bone). Releasing the tension in the muscle belly and tendons of the hip flexors likely reduces the compressive forces these muscles can exert on the lymphatic ducts that cross the hip region. With resolution of the muscle tension, the inflammatory products and the pent up fluid can then move out of the abdomen through the newly opened, decompressed ducts.

     Other muscles of note when gently digging for pelvic pain relief are deep-rooted external, or outward, hip rotators. The obturator internus and externus, and the superior and inferior gemelli muscles span deep across the pelvis and attach to the femur (thigh bone) on either side. These muscles appear to not only have the sinewy feel, but also a sense of guarding. Soft tissue mobilization (massage) and retraining of these muscles to contract then relax appropriately are both keys to restoring the muscles' integrity. A gradual increase in hip exercises with small marches, leg lifts out to each side, rotations inward and outward, and bridges can be easily implemented as home exercises once the patients grasp the correct techniques. (See Figure 34.) These exercises combined with a thorough stretching program can complement the hands-on mobilization of the muscles, ultimately restoring the muscles' normal resting tone and ability to work then relax when appropriate.

Figure 34. An illustration of a home exercise program to condition the hip muscles.

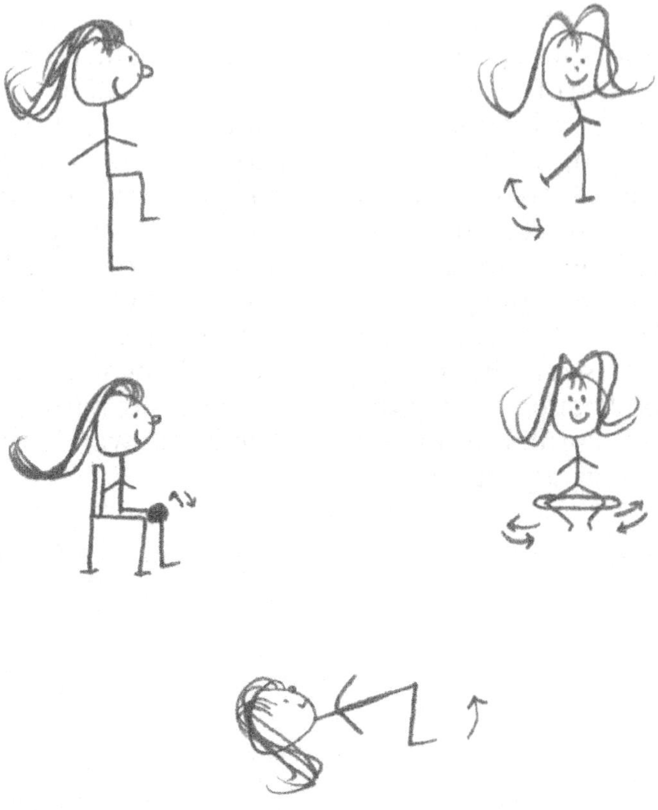

"Your hands are like magic!"

Shelly was a case that exemplified the power of manual soft tissue mobilization in the realm of pelvic inflammatory disorders and pelvic pain. Shelly repeatedly presented with inflammation in the abdomen and in thoracic and lumbar paraspinals (mid and low back muscles). Narcotics, diuretics, and a diet geared toward reducing bladder and endometrial inflammation did not do the trick. What was the magic potion? Hands-on therapy. Manually mobilizing the iliacus and iliopsoas muscles (hip flexors) drastically reduced her bladder pain, and the swelling in her abdomen and pelvic region ceased instantaneously. Thoracic, lumbar, and sacral (mid back, low back and just above the tailbone) soft tissue mobilization resolved her back pain and likely reduced any excessive tension on the nerves targeting the abdominal and pelvic contents. This occurred with **every single visit**. The patterns were the same, the treatments were the same, and the results were the same. And, after every visit, the patient would tell me, "Your hands are like magic! They make the swelling and the pain go away!"

Why did the pain repeatedly resume? I speculate it was the presence of a calcified mass. Describing her pain, the patient painted me a visual of a limestone-encrusted ball of stiff, sharp steel wool. The irritating mass likely scratched away at the internal abdominal wall, and possibly scratched the bladder, the uterus, the ligamentous structures, and the iliopsoas (hip flexor). I visualized scar tissue building as the tissues attempted to repair themselves, only to have that scar tissue torn at as well. Inflammation likely developed as the sheering and scratching continued.

In Shelly's case, a difficulty lay in the inability to

contract the transverse abdominis, which in other cases helped to hold a mass in place. Transverse abdominis contraction had helped Shelly with previous bouts of bladder pain, however, as the mass grew, the contraction of the transverse abdominis increased the tension and tugged on the region housing the mass. Therefore, we stopped attempting to contract the transverse abdominis and resorted to contracting only the pelvic floor for support. The Kegel did not increase the pain. With successive treatments, we curbed the inflammatory cycle by keeping the guarding at bay. The muscle tension that had compressed the abdominal contents and the nerves that controlled them was lifted.

    The hands-on soft tissue mobilization alleviated Shelly's pain when nothing else did. The increase in pelvic floor strength supported the pelvic contents allowing for mild to moderate activity without agitation. As of this writing, a surgery was scheduled for removal of the mass. In the mean time, physical therapy allowed Shelly to work and carry out life's necessary functions, and even to enjoy a stroll on the beach without excruciating pain.

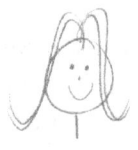

Every Little Bit of Pain Relief Helps

"...any amount of relief, large or small, is so very much appreciated."

In discussing with a patient her endometriosis, interstitial cystitis, and fibroids, I stated that I may not help to relieve all the pain that she had, but...and she interjected with the very words about to stream from my mouth, "...any amount of relief, large or small, is so very much appreciated."

Pelvic conditions are infamous for creating a domino effect of painful conditions. Pelvic pain often creates a myriad of secondary effects, but they can be treated successfully with physical therapy. With pelvic inflammation, muscle guarding in the iliopsoas (hip flexor) can ensue. Excessive anterior (forward) pelvic tilt can then over-extend the low back with a hyperlordotic curve. Such hyperlordosis (sway back) can irritate the spine's facet joints and the lumbar soft tissues, and push the lumbar intervertebral discs anteriorly or forward...and, the saga can continue. Minimizing the hip flexor tension can reduce the chances of the developing the successive conditions, and drastically alleviate pain. This is just one possible scenario, though. It is important for clinicians to seek out and catch as many of the proverbial dominoes as possible to help remove each layer of pain, to maximize the wellbeing of patients with pelvic disorders.

Furthermore, we must remember that despite always targeting the primary sources of the symptoms, we should treat the secondary conditions as well. The secondary conditions can mimic traumas that inflict a painful inflammatory response.[41] Therefore, in conjunction with managing the primary diagnoses of pelvic dysfunction and their own immediate painful manifestations, treating the secondary ailments can significantly reduce patients' *overall* pain. By resolving the secondary effects of an underlying inflammatory condition, we can immensely help restore patients' function despite the presence a pelvic disorder.

Please understand that my intent is **not** to treat **only** the symptoms. My intent is to treat the whole picture. Unfortunately the words, "There is no cure for endometriosis" continue to be fed to patients with this condition. Let's make it a mission in the rehabilitation process to let a woman *feel* like she does not have the condition, at least for short while. The power of positive thinking shines when a patient has pain relief for even a small period of time. The stress associated with pain is alleviated, as is stress's accomplice, cortisol. With small, progressive reductions in pain level, there is a growing ray of light at the end of the tunnel. I am not one to give false hope, but I **never** underestimate the power of the human body to rehabilitate. Treating painful inflammatory disorders of the pelvic region is fragile. However, every ounce of pain lifted allows a woman to enjoy life that much more.

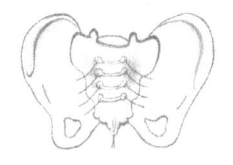

A Team Approach

Some pelvic disorders warrant a team of clinicians. With the knowledge of factors that interfere with recovery, clinicians can prompt patients to seek any and all of the necessary clinical team members. Interstitial cystitis and cortisol's effect on its associated bladder pain exemplify this point. As previously mentioned, cortisol is a hormone associated with stress responses. Lower levels of cortisol, which naturally occur in the morning time, appear to associate with greater bladder pain,[35] despite higher levels seeming to associate with painful bloating. Therefore, a balanced hormonal release appears to be needed in order to curb the pain and inflammation associated with interstitial cystitis. With knowledge of the underlying associations among hormones and provocations of pain and inflammation, clinicians can direct patients to specialists for appropriate testing and treatment, and educate patients on the many causes and treatments of such a condition.

It is important to emphasize that clinicians have a responsibility to point patients down the correct path for complete resolution of their diagnoses. These paths are the spokes of the wheel, and clinicians are at the hub. With a strong background in pelvic disorders, physical therapists can point patients in the most beneficial directions if physical therapy (physiotherapy) is not the only discipline necessary for successful recovery. The combined efforts of all clinicians involved can assist patients in achieving successful rehabilitation, exemplifying the importance of the holistic approach. If an impasse in recovery is reached with one means of treatment, guiding patients to another means improves overall care, eases patients' stress by giving them another avenue of hope, and speeds patients down the road to overall recovery.

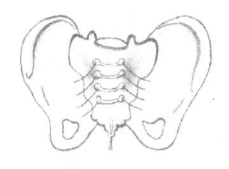

Pain with Emotional Stress is NOT Psychosomatic...

I Repeat,
Pain with Emotional Stress is NOT Psychosomatic

I am aware of online communities that are irate at the thought of pelvic pain being linked to emotional stress. My next section is by *no* means suggesting a psychosomatic nature to pelvic pain. However, *emotional stress can physically manifest* as muscle guarding, organ deficiency, menstrual irregularity, and unbearable pain.

Links between stress and physical increases in pain have not been solidified, but associations have been made. Stress and its accompanying release of the hormone cortisol have been linked to abdominal bloating, abdominal pain, back pain, and muscle tension. Heightened stress has also led to increases in heart rate and blood pressure, and has been linked to sleep disturbances and headaches. Cortisol can increase the production of inflammatory products. Inflammatory products can increase pain and swelling.[56] I am by no means stating that the pain associated with inflammatory disorders is solely stress-based. I am stating that stress can add to the pain and be a hindrance to healing, just as it can hinder the rehabilitation of back, neck, hip, shoulder, knee, ankle, and foot pain. I often tell my patients that stress finds pain and exacerbates it. With an elevated level of baseline pain, the release of cortisol can add fuel to the fire. The inflammatory products and swelling can hoist the existing pain level. Therefore, stress and its unwelcomed accompaniments *can increase* the pain level of and wreak havoc on existing pain-producing, inflammatory conditions. To diagnose and treat pelvic pain, the *whole persona* should be examined and treated, as is the case for *every* condition in *any* part of the body. This holistic approach should therefore address stress, as it may heighten the pain that already exists in association with patients' pelvic conditions.

There are patients who have endured sexual trauma and abuse that may have additional pelvic floor conditions. Muscle tension, inflammation, and organ dysfunction on top of the trauma can be unbearable to fathom. Vivid emotional anguish may compound the pain already inherent in diagnoses such as torn or repeatedly strained hip flexors, irritable bowel syndrome, interstitial cystitis, endometriosis, fibroids, and calcified masses. Emotional stress, in my opinion, can find the areas of vulnerability and attack them. The baseline of pain with organ dysfunction and with the presence of masses is already high. Adding emotional stress, with its release of cortisol and its snowballing cascade of painful responses, can kick that pain up a notch to a level deemed excruciating…rating a 12 on a scale from 1 to 10.

Post-traumatic stress disorder is alive in our communities. The stress associated with physical and mental trauma can manifest physically as pain and pain's accompaniments. The sources of all aspects of pain regardless of the condition must be identified in order to truly heal. Physical ailments incurred by a trauma, such as receiving a bullet wound, getting hit by a motor vehicle, being chased and beaten by a combat enemy, or being sexually abused, must be addressed. And, the emotional trauma of enduring such a horrific event simply cannot be overlooked. Patients' pain can stem from multiple sources. Each source contributes to the whole picture, and each source must be addressed in order to fully rehabilitate.

Stress can contribute to a number of physical conditions, such as heart disease, high blood pressure, and irritable bowel syndrome. It can also increase the pain of Crohn's disease and ulcerative colitis by contributing to flares.[56] Why, then, would it be difficult to accept stress as a contributor to or a source of *some* pain in *some* cases of pelvic pain? Pelvic pain stemming from vaginal childbirths, cesarean sections, fibroids, calcified masses, muscular and ligamentous disorders, lumbar disc displacements, menses, endometriosis, interstitial cystitis, cancer, physical abuse, sexual abuse, *and* from emotional trauma should *all* be treated in order to win the battle against pelvic pain. Some pain can stem from physical trauma, while some can stem from emotional trauma. All contributors must be overcome for that light at the end of the tunnel to keep getting brighter.

Exercise-induced endorphin release may help reduce stress and its physical manifestations of pain and painful inflammation. Exercise has been associated with a release of endorphins,[57] the 'feel good hormones'. These endorphins have been linked to reduced mental and emotional stress, and to reduced pain levels.[58] Endorphins have also been found to suppress cortisol production.[59] Performing physical exercise, such as walking or swimming, may therefore be beneficial to relieving patients' pain, stress, and stress's associated cortisol production and inflammatory response.

For some patients with pelvic pain, however, excessive jolting, as with some forms of exercise, can inflame tissues that are intertwined with calcified masses or fibroids. This jolting can create an abrasion of the tissues housing the masses. Exercise in these cases should be carefully selected and monitored so as to not create such abrasive forces on the tissues that are injured or are on the brink of further irritation. Furthermore, some patients may experience increased pain with exercise's addition of intra-abdominal pressure onto an already inflamed bladder or uterus. Physical therapists can help select the types of exercise that fit the patient's profile to promote endorphin release and overall health, while minimizing or preventing agitation.

Strong pelvic floor muscles can minimize the excursion of the tissues that sustain the jolt with exercise, helping patients exercise for overall health and achieve the endorphin release. This is an instance where physical therapy comes into play. Isolated pelvic floor exercise and core control can help maximize the ability to perform the activities that reduce stress and the pain it can create. If the pelvic floor is weak, its muscles should be gradually strengthened with an astute eye and ear to minimize detrimental over-fatigue. Over-fatigue, once again, can lessen the pelvic floor's abilities to render support and provide for continence with daily activities. Careful progression of isolated Kegels can allow the pelvic floor to best provide the necessary scaffolding and maintain continence while being strengthened. In addition to minimizing abrasion, holding pelvic contents in place, and providing continence, the pelvic floor is an integral component of the core, which holds the pelvis and spine in alignment while engaging in endorphin-releasing activities. A strong pelvic floor and full core (as long as the deep abdominal contraction does not irritate tissue housing a calcified mass) can help patients to engage in endorphin-releasing activities such as walking, running, swimming, hiking, cycling, weight lifting, surfing, and rock climbing to maximize stress and pain suppression, yet minimize agitation to an injured region.

[Note: Previously I mentioned that lower levels of cortisol were found to correlate with increased bladder pain in patients with interstitial cystitis.[35] Lowering the level of cortisol with exercise-induced endorphin release would then seem counterproductive to treating patients with interstitial cystitis. However, perhaps lowering the cortisol and its promotion of painful bloating on the bladder would make up for any pain created in the bladder. Endorphin's pain relieving properties may also negate the bladder pain incurred by cortisol suppression. Further research is needed to draw better conclusions.]

Core and isolated Kegel exercises may not only help to support the pelvis and the spine, they may also help to remove fluid pressure associated with bloating and inflammation. In some patients whose pain levels increase with emotional stress, tension can build in the stomach's trigger point beneath the sternum, and painful bloating can grow in the abdominal region. An increase in fluid retention may associate with stress's hormonal variations. Bloating and inflammation may be minimized with diet, with soft tissue mobilization (massage), and with Kegels and full core exercises. In cases such as these, asking patients to gently press on the stomach point can decompress the built-up tension. Asking them to lightly run their fingers along the external surfaces of the abdomen and pelvic cavity can reduce the region's surface tension. Kegels and core exercises can help to resolve stagnancy and painful cramping likely by increasing circulation in the pelvic and abdominal regions with a muscle pumping action. In addition, pressure on the bladder due to fluid retention in the abdomen can not only intensify bladder pain, it can also intensify urinary urgency. Countering the increased difficulty in holding urine makes the isolated Kegel yet again the pinnacle of successful continence. Physically removing the fluid pressure and countering its associated pain and urinary urgency are important ingredients in restoring patients' function. And, listening to the patients to determine a means of alleviating the stress and emotional anguish that provokes that fluid build up should not be overlooked as a golden key to recovery.

Some causes of stress may be as apparent as starting a new job, welcoming a new baby into life, caring for elderly family members, or grieving the loss of a loved one. Other cases may not be so apparent and require a very open ear. Such cases may involve those who have been molested, raped, or otherwise abused.

Stress release is important in the recovery from a workday. What happens when the workday lasts 24 hours? I have coined the term *Mom Syndrome* for mothers who often do not find time in their day or night to de-stress or exercise. Many feel guilty in doing so. Therefore it is important to help moms find a way to even take 15 minutes out of the day or night to carve in a little 'me time'. It is important to help mothers realize that at least 15 minutes of 'me time' is not inappropriate. On the contrary, such time to de-stress can rejuvenate them, giving them more energy to tackle the job of being a mother and making them better at what they do! This is not your average therapy, but the education and the self-help strategizing can assist in minimizing stress, which may be a cause of excess abdominal pressure and pain.

I have come across emotional release countless times while mobilizing patients' soft tissues. Holding stress in the abdominal and pelvic regions is quite common. A history of physical trauma to the region can punctuate such stress, adding a physical component to the emotional anguish. Some of my patients with emotional stress have presented with tension and its associated pain in the iliopsoas (hip flexor) muscle. Manual soft tissue mobilization similar to a pressure point massage has helped to alleviate the painful restrictions. Sometimes, as the stress harnessed in the muscles released, tears would stream down my patients' faces, not due to painful palpation, but due to the release of emotions. I would tell my patients to continue to cry, to not hold back, and to not be embarrassed. They stepped into my office for pain relief, and sometimes that relief would come with a release of emotions. Tension in the pelvic musculature can associate with pain. Releasing that pressure can manually take the pain away. The release of emotional anguish, though, can minimize the pain's return.

One such case involved the physical and emotional trauma of a rape. The physical injuries as well as the guilt of having had intercourse, albeit forced and completely unintentional, with a man other than her husband were harnessed in Grace's pelvic region. Grace's lower thoracic and lumbar (mid and low back) and hip flexor muscles were restricted causing hyperlordosis (sway back). The right iliopsoas (hip flexor) being tighter than the left pulled the right ilium (side of pelvis) into anterior (forward) rotation. Grace was unable to contract her pelvic floor muscles for longer than 3 seconds likely due to the asymmetrical alignment's disadvantageous lengthening of the pelvic floor's muscle fibers. Having intercourse with her husband was painfully out of the question. In my opinion, emotional anguish and physically traumatic pain were all embedded in Grace's iliopsoas (hip flexor) and pelvic floor muscles. While administering light, grade 2 soft tissue mobilization (massage) to the iliopsoas, tears streamed down her face. Soon thereafter, Grace revealed the trauma in detail.

    With a series of physical therapy visits, Grace's physical and emotional traumas began to resolve. Grace performed *lava flow* exercises with a *'blow when you go'* breathing technique which gradually released the pelvic floor's painfully guarded contraction. Progressive soft tissue mobilization (massage) of the right iliopsoas (hip flexor) complemented right hip extension isometrics. Together the soft tissue release and isometric exercise corrected the forward rotation of the right ilium (side of pelvis). The hyperlordosis (sway back) resolved as soft tissue mobilization (massage) released the tension harnessed in the lumbar and thoracic paraspinals (low and mid back muscles) and iliopsoas (hip flexor) muscles. After 2 weeks, Grace was pain free and was able to enjoy intercourse with her husband. Resolving the physical strain and listening to Grace reveal her inner pain let her tension unravel and her healing begin. Although emotional healing from her devastating trauma was likely not complete, a barrier was broken and at least a part of her was freed.

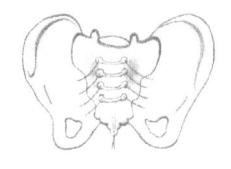

A Few More Words on Sexual Trauma

I speculate that sexual trauma can create a heightened level of tension due to a reactionary guarding of the pelvic floor muscles. Tension in the low back and hip flexor muscles may also increase, possibly due to positioning, pain response, and actual guarding during the attack. A hit in the nose can cause facial muscles to swell. A blunt trauma to the arm or thigh can provoke swelling and muscle guarding. Scraping the roof of the mouth can cause soreness and swelling. Sexual attacks can cause pain, swelling, and muscle guarding. It is important to see sexual trauma as indeed a *trauma* with the repercussions of such. A means to reduce inflammation, restore mobility, and restore use of the surrounding musculature are all needed for rehabilitation to be complete. A fear of getting hit by a car after a motor vehicle accident may cause a flinching at the thought or sight of a quickly approaching automobile. Such a guarding response can increase tension and pain, and can reduce mobility. A sexual trauma can instill fear, cause flinching, and cause muscle guarding as well. Therefore, the sexual trauma may have physical characteristics due to physical injury as well as emotional pain that physically manifests and adds to tension to the pelvic region.

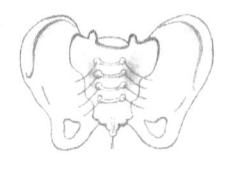

Overcoming Emotional Stress as Sexual Abuse Survivor: Step Outside of Yourself to Treat Yourself

I am going out on a limb here in this next section, but it is for good reason. I do not pretend to be a psychologist or psychiatrist, but I have a background in the psychological arena having studied under world-renowned psychologists at Yale and having listened to my patients as they overcame incredibly traumatic experiences. The emotional stress associated with a sexual trauma or otherwise inflicted abuse is a delicate subject. I understand the connection of emotions and physical presentation and have helped several people work through emotional stress while assisting them in recovering from the physical trauma. I have worked with patients that have overcome the physical barriers of pain as well as the stagnant emotions tied up in the pelvic region.

As cliché as it sounds, oftentimes what it takes to understand a hardship is going through a similar ordeal. Several patients have studied abuse traumas similar to their own. Some have even helped others overcome theirs. But overcoming one's own afflictions is a challenging task. So I ask my patients to step outside themselves to become the healer, in order to release the anguish plaguing the person in the mirror's reflection.

I speculate that the difficulty in trying to understand *how* and *why* abuse happened is often harnessed in the hip flexors' tension, the pelvic floor's tension, and in the knot in the stomach's trigger point. For patients who have endured abuse *and have other pelvic diagnoses*, the *how* and *why* may be embedded in the endometriotic and scar tissues of the uterus, the scar tissues encompassing the calcified masses, the inflamed detrusor muscle of the bladder, and in any other weakened pelvic organ. With or without other conditions of pelvic dysfunction, standing erect, walking upstairs, and taking a deep breath are all painful when emotional stress grips and restricts movement in tissues and organs. The physical pain sustained while having intercourse with a loved one makes the lovemaking unbearable. Racking the brain to figure how and why the abuse occurred can add to an emotional overload and to the pain that follows.

It can be difficult for a patient to disclose the abuse, and it can be even more difficult and frustrating to teach someone else to understand its effects. These frustrations only add to the emotional frenzy and the pain. Therefore, the best healer may be the patient. I will now speak directly to the patients in my audience, but clinicians, partners, and family members, please hear my words to the patients. If you are frustrated in making verbal sense of an experience because you do not think the listening ear comprehends, you are quite possibly correct. It is time to become your own healer. If you were to listen to another victim of your very own devastation, what would you tell him or her? Answer that question and you will start to heal yourself. Step outside yourself and see where you are emotionally, then use your experience to guide yourself to recovery. Sometimes it takes words, tears, rages of anger, trips to far away lands, climbing tall mountains, or setting new goals for yourself. But ultimately the healing begins with self-discovery, telling yourself as your own healer that the physical abuse is in the past, and that you are above the experience and the perpetrator. Looking at and listening to yourself from the outside just may give rise to your ability to heal yourself, and that healing may begin with an understanding of what is truly the source of your emotional pain. The physical attack tragically took a part of you. Don't let the emotional anguish take the rest. Instead of trying to make someone else understand, step outside yourself as the victim, listen to yourself, and become your own healer.

    For patients overcoming abuse who have also experienced dyspareunia (painful intercourse): When in a relationship, it is important to understand and let your partner understand that the emotional and physical anguish of abuse can periodically rear its ugly head. Even if the pain subsides enough for intercourse at one point, that pain can surface again, though hopefully to a lesser degree. The pain may render intercourse unbearable. Remember, though, that intimacy manifests in many forms. Getting creative with intimacy integrates your partner into the healing process. That integration draws a closeness that just may keep the painful tension from striking so often, or ever again.

    I would now like to speak to the patients' sexual partners. Clinicians, family members and patients, please hear my words to the partners. When your partner's pain with intercourse has subsided and regular intercourse has begun, it is of utmost importance for you to state when and why you are at a lull in sexual desire. Sexually shunning the victim can, on some occasions, set the victim into an emotional tailspin with feelings of rejection, tensing the pelvic floor and making intercourse very painful. Patients, I would advise explaining this possible scenario to your partners. Openly communicating why and when a sexual pattern takes a downward turn are important for both parties, especially when one of the parties is a victim of sexual assault.

Stepping outside oneself to treat oneself is not an easy task. Understanding what the problems are does not necessarily dictate how to treat them. To those who are willing to give it a shot, take a deep breath and get ready for the plunge. The breath you take on the other side will be most refreshing.

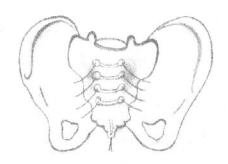

In Overcoming Anguish of a Trauma, Sometimes Forgiveness is Not the Answer

My next words may offend some readers, and for any offense taken I apologize in advance. But, I could not exclude what I am about to say. For those who take offense, please remember we are all unique in our means of healing. What I am about to say has helped more than just a handful of my patients...

The limb onto which I will now venture reaches into a patient's spirituality. Amidst the release of physical tension, the balancing of muscle strength surrounding the torso, and the strengthening of the pelvic floor, spirituality is often overlooked. Spirituality, in every amount from nil to abundant, is part of a patient's whole being and is strongly considered in my holistic treatment.

Time and time again I have heard that forgiving a wrongdoing will set one free from emotional anguish. With this piece of advice is the caveat that the forgiveness does not excuse the "wrongdoer", it releases the victim from the emotional pain associated with the wrongdoing. While this gesture may work for some victims, I disagree that it is a universal mantra. I will proudly state that is not necessary to "forgive" a rapist, a molester, or an abuser of any caliber. What the offender did is not okay. It was a complete wrongdoing. The offender does not necessarily need to be excused or pardoned for healing to occur. In speaking with patients of sexual abuse, especially those who were afflicted as children, one of the hardest ideas to comprehend is the act of forgiving a person who acted so selfishly and maliciously against them. I will go against the status quo and say, "It is okay not to forgive…"

When speaking these words to patients, I have often received a perplexed, yet relieved look and an emphatic "thank you". The anguish associated with trauma is more than one ever deserves. Trying to forgive the wrongdoing sometimes adds fuel to the emotional fire. I would like to state that it is absolutely 'okay' to rise above the norm and absolutely not forgive an abuser. Relinquishing the notion that forgiveness is the answer is freeing and empowering, and may be the chisel one needs to start tearing down the literal and figurative walls of pent up pain.

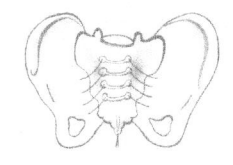

A Few Words Specifically for Men!

Having treated many men with pelvic floor concerns over the years, I have found tips that I would like to share! Several of the men that I have treated presented with prostate enlargement, with trouble controlling urinary flow. Learning to integrate long Kegels and quick agility Kegels into their daily activities, and learning to fully release the bladder contents with the *blow when you go* technique helped these patients gain control of leakage and urgency, and achieve improved voids. For those opting for surgical removal of the prostate, a dose of *blowing when going* and learning to control the Kegel muscles *before* surgery helped before and dramatically *after* surgery! After surgery, sensing urinary leakage *and* sensing the whereabouts of the pelvic floor muscles can be difficult. Those two sensation deficiencies together can add up to an incontinent disaster! Furthermore, pelvic floor muscle guarding after prostate surgery can wreak havoc on the ability to fully void. Incomplete voids, as stated previously, can lead to urinary urgency. Without the ability to find and hold the Kegel muscles, incontinence can thusly ensue. Patients who learn pelvic floor control techniques before surgery often find it much easier to gain or regain control of the pelvic floor post-operatively than those who do not. Take home messages? Learning how to Kegel and release can help combat prostate pressures, and if surgery is in the cards, learning to do so beforehand can make the road to recovery an easier one!

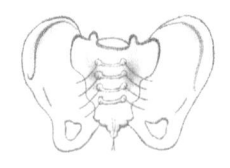

Disorders Involving Control of the Pelvic Floor, Without a Drop of Incontinence

In the game of life, the pelvic floor is often the MVP. Sometimes pelvic floor weakness is overlooked as a contributor to a condition because the patient does not have a trace of incontinence. What is lacking, though, is the strength needed to assist the rest of the core in stabilizing the trunk.

By her early thirties, Kalea had endured a 10-year history of lumbar (low back), pelvic, and sacroiliac joint instability. As previously described, the sacroiliac joint is where the lower part of the spine, above the tailbone, meets the pelvis. She presented with elevation and anterior (forward) rotation of the right ilium (side of pelvis). Kalea reported an inability to sit or stand for more than five minutes without excruciating pain. She had previously seen four separate physical therapists, who all improved upon her symptoms while in she was in therapy, but offered no lasting effects of the treatments. The piece of the puzzle that was missing was the incorporation of the pelvic floor with lumbar-pelvic and sacroiliac (low back, pelvic, and sacral) stabilization. Upon evaluation, Kalea could not contract the pelvic floor voluntarily, but she could automatically hold urine when she had the urge to void. Here is a classic case of the importance of increasing the control of the pelvic floor muscles for spinal and sacroiliac joint stabilization. Use of 50 Hz electrical vaginal stimulation while Kegeling in supine, then in sitting, then in standing, and then with walking allowed Kalea to progressively stabilize the low back, pelvic, and sacral joints with improved pelvic floor muscle control. With time and practice, Kalea was able to incorporate the Kegel into her daily activities improving her overall function. Pelvic floor training was an integral part of therapy, other components being soft tissue mobilization (massage) for tension release in the lumbar paraspinals (low back muscles) and hip flexors, body mechanics training, and transverse abdominis (deep abdominal muscle) conditioning. All together, the rehabilitative puzzle pieces allowed Kalea to not only stand and sit, but to bike and walk long distances, and even hike on uneven surfaces without exacerbations of painful low back, pelvic, and sacral instability.

Despite no trace of incontinence, pelvic floor strengthening was still the link to improving Kalea's functioning. Without pelvic floor strength, the trunk's core was not stabilized. Without stability throughout the core, painful joint malalignments disrupted an otherwise pleasant stroll on the beach. By specifically targeting the pelvic floor, the full core could engage. Strongly contracting the full core gave Kalea her best shot at minimizing recurring episodes of painful instability.

A similar need to the strengthen the pelvic floor presented in 53 year-old Lindsay with a 10-year history of left hip and low back pain stemming from severe osteoarthritis. She had been lacking the use of her core, specifically the use of her pelvic floor muscles. She presented with left ilial (side of pelvis) elevation in correlation with significant tension in the left lumbar (low back) soft tissues, particularly the quadratus lumborum.

Despite using techniques to repeatedly bring the pelvis to its pain-free level, the pelvis needed stabilization. The missing link to Lindsay's stabilization, like Kalea's, was a strong contraction of the pelvic floor.

Overuse of low back muscles has created an imbalance of tension and an unfavorable pelvic alignment in many of my patients. This I cannot overstate! The quadratus lumborum and other low back muscles can be used to move the spine, and to stabilize the spine when resisting an oncoming force. When an outfielder catches a line drive, the lumbar muscles may resist the rotation of the trunk that is inherent in stopping an object moving at mach speed. A canoe paddler recruits the low back muscles to propel her across the ocean. When the pelvic floor is weak, however, these same low back muscles (which attach onto the buttocks region) are also often recruited to keep the pelvis, sacrum, and coccyx (all in the area of the buttocks region) in alignment. The low back muscles can then become overworked from compensating for a core weakened by a lackadaisical pelvic floor. Overtaxing these outer muscles can generate tension responsible for a wrongful tugging on the pelvis. Asymmetrical pull can create the infamous ilial (side of pelvis) elevation. Release of the low back muscle tension often requires the application of soft tissue mobilization (massage). Once the tension subsides, stretching the ilium in a downward motion can align the pelvis. (The side of the pelvis that is elevated is stretched downward to level the sides of the pelvis. See previous Figure 16.) Such alignment can eventually be stabilized with strong core strengthening, incorporating the pelvic floor. I previously presented this scenario in discussing many a patient with incontinence and strain of the pelvic floor musculature. In those cases, the malalignment was both a cause and a result of pelvic floor weakness. In this section, I am presenting cases whereby the pelvic floor weakness is not contributing to incontinence, but *is* generating painful joint destabilization and calling upon other muscles to overwork and pick up its slack!

Stella was diagnosed with hip degeneration, with a possible tear in the labrum. The labrum resembles a suction cup functioning to hold the hip joint in place. Her pain seemed to stem from compression of the femoral-acetabular (hip) joint caused by severely restricted muscles that crossed it. What had caused this muscle tension? My speculation is that a weakened pelvic floor recruited the use of the hip flexors, hip extensors, and hip rotators to work overtime in supporting the spine and pelvic region, giving them minimal recovery. Lacking stretches in her daily regime, the hip rotators, extensors, and flexors likely shortened with tension and harshly pulled the hip joint into a compressed state, giving the head of the femur (thigh bone) no choice but to grind in the acetabulum where it met the pelvis. This grinding likely pushed and tugged on the labrum and created pain within the joint. On the road to surgery, Stella detoured into my office and realized the importance of the pelvic floor's role of trunk stability and hip integrity. Her labrum was not torn. Her pain subsided as the pelvic floor muscles strengthened and the hip muscles released their painfully excessive grip on the hip joint.

Without trunk stability generated in large part by a strong pelvic floor, the hips can assume the sheering forces of a bobbling torso and endure brutally painful compression. The hip muscles may be called upon to compensate for a slacking pelvic floor and become tense with overexertion. Once Stella received therapy to improve the contraction timing and strength of the pelvic floor muscles and to reduce the tension in the muscles crossing the hip joint, she noted remarkable improvements in her function and pain level. Stella was eventually able to incorporate Kegels into her daily activities, making the contraction of the pelvic floor muscles more automatic. With the incorporation of small pelvic tilts and 'fidgeting' for circulation, Stella was able to sit for four hours in work meetings without pain. With a combination of pelvic floor muscle strengthening, body mechanics training, soft tissue mobilization (massage), and gradual progression of hip and trunk conditioning, Stella realized she did not need a hip replacement. The key player once again was a stronger pelvic floor, this time ridding the need for compensatory muscle recruitment and halting that recruitment's detriment to the hip joints.

In summary, just because a patient does not have incontinence does not mean the pelvic floor is in the utmost shape. Overlooking the pelvic floor as a contributor to trunk and hip diagnoses could send a patient into unnecessary surgery or onto unnecessary pain medications. Careful dissection of the patient's full presentation once again bodes well for successful rehabilitation.

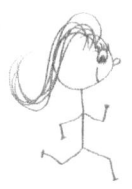

In Conclusion...

The importance and intricacy of pelvic health in the scope of physical therapy practice is immense. Treatment of the pelvic region reaches well beyond the diagnoses of prolapses, spasms, inflammations, complications with childbirth, and incontinence. It provides a foundation, a scaffold, and a figurative life support getting patients back in the game we call life.

Enlightening patients on the commonalities among many women handling pelvic dysfunction eases the stress associated with having these conditions. By making it known that there are many, many people who have overcome pelvic disorders, I hope to make seeking help a little easier. One of my goals as the author of this book is to open discussions about conditions that may be embarrassing to share or are thought to be untreatable or incurable. Sharing treatment techniques is another. With open communication and an open mind, conditions that are holding patients hostage can be conquered. Those very patients can return to a life without embarrassment, without pain, and without bulky undergarments!

Thank you for affording me the opportunity to share the knowledge I have gained from my patients and through my research. I hope to have provided you, my audience, with the notion that pelvic dysfunction is vastly common and can be helped. Please spread the word that pelvic disorders are at least treatable if not curable with conservative measures and self-help techniques. Trust me, thousands of future patients that surround you will be thankful you did! Not only can overcoming pelvic dysfunction erase an illness from a medical chart, it can bring a patient back to life.

Epilogue

As my first edition book went to print, with excerpts from my book, I voyaged to a nation plagued by pelvic dysfunction. Since writing a paper for an anthropology class as an undergraduate at Yale, I have been determined to provide rehabilitation assistance to women of Africa afflicted by torturous cultural practices. As if the cultural practice of genital mutilation is not traumatic enough, adding childbirth to an already devastated pelvic region makes incontinence a common occurrence. Even without childbirth, intercourse for women with immense scar tissue and other complications is traumatic to the pelvic floor. Incontinence for these women is not only a wet nuisance during their daily activities, it is also considered grounds for ostracizing them from their communities. Mutilated, scarred, and ostracized. For the time being at least, my opinion of female genital mutilation will be left at home. My mission in Africa is not to step on cultural toes, although I would like to stomp on a few! My goal is to teach women how to gain control of the pelvic floor. In doing so, I hope to spread the training from generation to generation. Just as teaching one man or woman to fish feeds a village, teaching one woman to control her pelvic floor keeps generations continent, and welcome in their communities.

References

[1] Herschorn S MD, FRCSC. Female Pelvic Floor Anatomy: The Pelvic Floor, Supporting Structures, and Pelvic Organs. Rev Urol. 2004; 6(Suppl 5): S2–S10. Retrieved via http://www.ncbi.nlm.nih.gov/pmc/articles/PMC1472875/. August 23, 2014.

[2] Guaderrama NM1, Liu J, Nager CW, Pretorius DH, Sheean G, Kassab G, Mittal RK. Evidence for the Innervation Of Pelvic Floor Muscles By The Pudendal Nerve. Journal Obstet Gynecol. 2005 Oct;106(4):774-81. Retrieved via http://www.ncbi.nlm.nih.gov/pubmed/16199635. August 22, 2014.

[3] Todd LT Jr, Yaszemski MJ, Currier BL, Fuchs B, Kim CW, Sim FH. Bowel And Bladder Function After Major Sacral Resection. Clin Orthop Relat Res. 2002 Apr;(397):36-9. Retrieved via http://www.ncbi.nlm.nih.gov/pubmed/11953593. August 23, 2014.

[4] Purves D, Augustine GJ, Fitzpatrick D, et al., editors. Neuroscience. 2nd edition. Sunderland (MA): Sinauer Associates; 2001. N pag. Retrieved via http://www.ncbi.nlm.nih.gov/books/NBK10886/. August 24, 2014

[5] Kegel AH MD, F.A.C.S. A Nonsurgical Method of Increasing the Tone of Sphincters and their Supporting Structures. 1948. Symposium presentation: Stress Incontinence and Genital Relaxation. CIBA Clinical Symposia, Feb-Mar 1952, Vol. 4, No. 2, pages 35-52. Retrieved via http://www.dothekegel.com/arnie/. August 23, 2014.

[6] http://www.health.harvard.edu/fhg/updates/update0805c.shtml. Retrieved October 1, 2014.

[7] http://my.clevelandclinic.org/services/urology-kidney/diseases-conditions/vaginal-prolapse. Retrieved October 1, 2014.

[8] http://www.hccfl.edu/media/383453/ch_25_summary.doc. Retrieved August 23, 2014.

[9] Fowler CJ, Griffiths D, de Groat WC. The Neural Control of Micturition. Nat Rev Neurosci. 2008 Jun; 9(6): 453–466. doi: 10.1038/nrn2401. Retrieved via http://www.ncbi.nlm.nih.gov/pmc/articles/PMC2897743/. October 1, 2014.

[10] Bø K, Talseth T, Holme I. Single Blind, Randomized Controlled Trial of Pelvic Floor Exercises, Electrical Stimulation, Vaginal Cones, and No Treatment In Management of Genuine Stress Incontinence In Women. BMJ. 1999 Feb 20;318(7182):487-93. Retrieved via http://www.ncbi.nlm.nih.gov/pubmed/10024253. August 24, 2014.

[11] Yamanishi T, Yasuda K, Sakakibara R, Hattori T, Ito H, Murakami S. Pelvic Floor Electrical Stimulation in the Treatment of Stress Incontinence: An Investigational Study and a Placebo Controlled Double-Blind Trial. J Urol. 1997 Dec;158(6):2127-31. Retrieved via http://www.ncbi.nlm.nih.gov/pubmed/9366328. August 24, 2014.

[12] Davila GW, Ghoniem GM, Wexner SD. Pelvic Floor Dysfunction: A Multidisciplinary Approach. Springer Science & Business Media, 2008 Dec 23; page 175, with credits to Joanna M. Togami and Gamal M. Ghoniem. Retrieved via http://books.google.com/books?id=fvXo3tPTnO8C&printsec=frontcover#v=onepage&q&f=false. December 24, 2014.

[13] http://michaeldmann.net/mann14.html. N pag. Retrieved on December 25, 2014

[Please note that information on this topic was also found at the following site, but the information was no longer available online as of December 24, 2014.
http://ab.mec.edu/abrhs/science/anatphys_labs/backgroundlengthtension.html . Retrieved October 15, 2014.]

[14] Wreje U, Kristiansson P, Aberg H, Byström B, von Schoultz B. Serum Levels of Relaxin during the Menstrual Cycle and Oral Contraceptive Use. Gynecol Obstet Invest. 1995;39(3):197-200. Retrieved via http://www.ncbi.nlm.nih.gov/pubmed/7789917. May 14, 2014

[15] Ferguson KL, McKey PL, Bishop KR, Kloen P, Verheul JB, Dougherty MC. Stress Urinary Incontinence: Effect of Pelvic Muscle Exercise. Obstet Gynecol. 1990 Apr;75(4):671-5. Retrieved via http://www.ncbi.nlm.nih.gov/pubmed/2314786. August 24, 2014.

[16] Sherman RA, Davis GD, Wong MF. Behavioral Treatment of Exercise-Induced Urinary Incontinence Among Female Soldiers. Mil Med. 1997

Oct;162(10):690-4. Retrieved via http://www.ncbi.nlm.nih.gov/pubmed/9339085. September 17, 2014.

[17] Pelvic Floor Muscle Training Exercises. Kegel Exercises. A.D.A.M. Medical Encyclopedia. Last reviewed: June 18, 2012. N pag. Retrieved via http://www.nlm.nih.gov/medlineplus/ency/article/003975.htm. September 17, 2014.

[18] Price N, Dawood R, Jackson SR. Pelvic Floor Exercise for Urinary Incontinence: A Systematic Literature Review. Department of Obstetrics and Gynaecology, John Radcliffe Hospital, Oxford OX3 9DU, UK. Review accepted August 10, 2010. N pag. Retrieved via http://www.oxfordgynaecology.com/Publications/Pelvic%20floorexercisefor urinaryincontinenceAsystematicliteraturereview.pdf. November 19, 2014.

[19] Teleman PM, Persson J, Mattiasson A, Samsioe G. The Relation between Urinary Incontinence and Steroid Hormone Levels in Perimenopausal Women. A report from the Women's Health in the Lund Area (WHILA) Study. Acta Obstet Gynecol Scand. 2009;88(8):927-32. doi: 10.1080/00016340903117986. Retrieved via http://www.ncbi.nlm.nih.gov/pubmed/19679140. September 17, 2014.

[20] https://embryology.med.unsw.edu.au/embryology/index.php/File:Menstrual _cycle.png. N pag. Retrieved December 25, 2014.

[21] Yamanishi T, Kamai T, Yoshida, K-I. Neuromodulation for the treatment of urinary incontinence. International Journal of Urology (2008) 15, 665–672 doi: 10.1111/j.1442-2042.2008.02080.x Review Article. Retrieved via http://www.imedicare.co.uk/media/50327/yamanishi_2008_review.pdf. December 25, 2014.

[Please note information on this topic was also found at the following site, but the information was no longer available online as of December 25, 2014: http://brazjurol.com.br/july_august_2013/Schereiner_454_464.pdf. Retrieved November 19, 2014.]

[22] Finazzi-Agrò E. et al. Percutaneous Tibial Nerve Stimulation (PTNS) in the Treatment of Urge Incontinence: A Double Blind Placebo Controlled Study. Poster, SIUD National Congress, Italy. (2005). N. pag. Retrieved via www.uroplasty.com/common/data/view/183#sthash.IMviez.dpuf. August 23, 2014.

[23] Bosch JL, Groen J. Sacral. (S3) Segmental Nerve Stimulation as a Treatment for Urge Incontinence in Patients with Detrusor Instability: Results of Chronic Electrical Stimulation Using an Implantable Neural Prosthesis. J Urol. 1995 Aug;154(2 Pt 1):504-7. Retrieved via http://www.ncbi.nlm.nih.gov/pubmed/7609117. August 23, 2014.

[24] Smith AL, Leung J, Kun S, Zhang R, Karagiannides I, Raz S, Lee U, Glovatscka V, Pothoulakis C, Bradesi S, Mayer EA, Rodríguez LV. The Effects of Acute and Chronic Psychological Stress on Bladder Function in a Rodent Model. Urology. 2011 Oct;78(4):967.e1-7. doi: 10.1016/j.urology.2011.06.041. Epub 2011 Aug 24. Retrieved via http://www.ncbi.nlm.nih.gov/pmc/articles/PMC3190050/. August 23, 2014.

[25] Dorsher PT, McIntosh, PM, Gleitman H, Fridlund AJ, Reisberg, D. Neurogenic Bladder. Psychology (6 ed.). W. W. Norton & Company. ISBN 0-393-97767-6. Adv Urol. 2012; 2012: 816274. Published online 2012 February 8. doi: 10.1155/2012/816274. Calm Clinic via www. April 4, 2013. N pag. Retrieved via Web September 17, 2014, no longer available as of December 25, 2014.

[26] Wood SK, Baez MA, Bhatnagar S, Valentino RJ. Social Stress-Induced Bladder Dysfunction: Potential Role of Corticotropin-Releasing Factor. Am J Physiol Regul Integr Comp Physiol. 2009 May;296(5):R1671-8. doi: 10.1152/ajpregu.91013.2008. Epub 2009 Mar 11. Retrieved via http://ajpregu.physiology.org/content/ajpregu/296/5/R1671.full.pdf. September 17, 2014.

[27] Sellers DJ, Chess-Williams R. Muscarinic Agonists and Antagonists: Effects on the Urinary Bladder. Handb Exp Pharmacol. 2012;(208):375-400. doi: 10.1007/978-3-642-23274-9_16. Retrieved via http://www.medscape.com/medline/abstract/22222707. September 17, 2014.

[28] Bogner, HR. M.D., M.S.C.E,a,b, O Donnell, AJ B.A,a,b, de Vries, HF M.S.P.H,a,b, Northington, GM M.D., PhD,c, Joo, JH M.D., M.AdJ. The Temporal Relationship between Anxiety Disorders and Urinary Incontinence among Community-Dwelling Adults Anxiety Disord. J Anxiety Disord. 2011 March; 25(2): 203–208. Published online 2010 September 17. doi: 10.1016/j.janxdis.2010.09.003 Retrieved via http://www.ncbi.nlm.nih.gov/pmc/articles/PMC3031666/. September 17, 2014.

[29] Durocher JJ, Klein JC, Carter JR. Attenuation of Sympathetic Baroreflex Sensitivity During the Onset of Acute Mental Stress in Humans. Am J Physiol Heart Circ Physiol. May 2011; 300(5): H1788–H1793. Published online Feb 25, 2011. doi: 10.1152/ajpheart.00942.2010. Retrieved via http://www.ncbi.nlm.nih.gov/pmc/articles/PMC3094089/. December 25, 2014.

[29b] Newman, D.K. (2002). New treatment options for overactive bladder and incontinence. The Director, 10(3).

[30] Bergland C. Cortisol: Why "The Stress Hormone" Is Public Enemy No. 1. The Athlete's Way, Sweat and the Biology of Bliss. 2013 Jan 22. N pag. Retrieved via http://www.psychologytoday.com/blog.the-atheletes-way. August 23, 2014.

[31] McMurray RG, Kocher PL, Horvath SM. Aerobic Power and Body Size Affects the Exercise-Induced Stress Hormone Responses to Varying Water Temperatures. Aviation Space and Environmental Medicine 1994;65(9 I):809-814. Retrieved via http://www.military-nutrition.com/Document/Publication/27982655?expertId=106. August 23, 2014.

[32] Hill EE, Zack E, Battaglini C, Viru M, Viru A, Hackney AC. Exercise and Circulating Cortisol Levels: The Intensity Threshold Effect. J Endocrinol Invest. 2008 Jul;31(7):587-91. Retrieved via http://www.ncbi.nlm.nih.gov/pubmed/18787373?ordinalpos=1&itool=Entrez System2.PEntr. August 23, 2014.

[33] http://my.clevelandclinic.org/health/diseases_conditions/hic_Bladder_Irritating_Foods. N paag. Retrieved August 23, 2014.

[34] Petropoulou O, Koumousidis A, Katsetos C, Varras M, Katsoulis M. Pathophysiological and Hormonal Changes Affecting Pain during Pregnancy: A Review. OA Women's Health 2013 Jun 01;1(1):5. Retrieved via http://www.oapublishinglondon.com/article/658. August 23, 2014.

[35] V. Chantarasorn and H. P. Dietz. Diagnosis of Cystocele Type by Clinical Examination and Pelvic Floor Ultrasound. Obstet Gynecol 2012; 39: 710–714. Wiley Online Library. DOI: 10.1002/uog.10156. Retrieved via http://onlinelibrary.wiley.com/doi/10.1002/uog.10156/full. October 30, 2014.

[36] Steensma AB, Oom DM, Burger CW, Schouten WR. Assessment of Posterior Compartment Prolapse: A Comparison of Evacuation Proctography and 3D Transperineal Ultrasound. Colorectal Dis. 2010 Jun;12(6):533-9. doi: 10.1111/j.1463-1318.2009.01936.x. Retrieved via https://books.google.com/books?id=IuugRTCHauMC&pg=PA144&lpg=PA144&dq=Assessment+of+posterior+compartment+prolapse:+a+comparison+of+evacuation+proctography+and+3D+transperineal+ultrasound.&source=bl&ots=Xl2SrQtRZM&sig=ni4Y86wxH2-8iCrVzCzR8y_R_eg&hl=en&sa=X&ei=Ry-dVPGpFozpoASF-oCQCQ&ved=0CDgQ6AEwBQ#v=onepage&q=Assessment%20of%20posterior%20compartment%20prolapse%3A%20a%20comparison%20of%20evacuation%20proctography%20and%203D%20transperineal%20ultrasound.&f=false. November 19, 2014.

[37] Thakar R, Sultan AH, Stankiewicz A. Accuracy of Assessing Pelvic Organ Prolapse Quantification Points Using Dynamic 2D Transperineal Ultrasound in Women with Pelvic Organ Pr. N pag. Retrieved via https://books.google.com/books?id=SUm4AQAAQBAJ&pg=PA88&dq=Thakar+R,+Sultan+AH,+Stankiewicz+A.+Accuracy+of+Assessing+Pelvic+Organ+Prolapse+Quantification+Points+Using+Dynamic+2D+Transperineal+Ultrasound+in+Women+with+Pelvic+Organ+Pr&hl=en&sa=X&ei=aTCdVNj-B4KLoQSA_oGoAw&ved=0CCEQ6AEwAA#v=onepage&q=Thakar%20R%2C%20Sultan%20AH%2C%20Stankiewicz%20A.%20Accuracy%20of%20Assessing%20Pelvic%20Organ%20Prolapse%20Quantification%20Points%20Using%20Dynamic%202D%20Transperineal%20Ultrasound%20in%20Women%20with%20Pelvic%20Organ%20Pr&f=false. October 30, 2014.

[38] Lexicographers: Anderson DM MA, Jefferson K MA, Novak PD PhD, Pronunciation Editor: Elliot MA BA. Dorland's Illustrated Medical Dictionary 28th Edition. W.B. Saunders Company, a Division of Harcourt Brace & Company. Philadelphia, 1994. Pgs 356, 1790. Print.

[39] Naqaish T, Rizvi F, Khattak JI. Impact of Kegel Exercise on Brink Scale and Activities of Daily Life (ADLs) in Patients of Cystocele. Journal of Rawalpindi Medical College (JRMC); 2013;17(2):243-246. Retrieved via http://www.journalrmc.com/volumes/1395218159.pdf. December 26, 2014.

[40] Bent AE, MD. Sling and Bulking Agent Placement Procedures Rev. Urol. 2004; 6(Suppl 5): S26–S46. Retrieved via http://www.ncbi.nlm.nih.gov/pmc/articles/PMC1472872/. August 23, 2104.

[41] http://www.nlm.nih.gov/medlineplus/ency/article/000821.htm. Retrieved September 17, 2014.

[42] www.physioworks.com.au. Retrieved September 7, 2015.

[43] Wreje U, Kristiansson P, Aberg H, Byström B, von Schoultz B. Serum Levels of Relaxin during the Menstrual Cycle and Oral Contraceptive Use. Gynecol Obstet Invest. 1995;39(3):197-200. Retrieved via http://www.ncbi.nlm.nih.gov/pubmed/7789917. Retrieved September 17, 2014.

[44] http://www.ncbi.nlm.nih.gov/pubmedhealth/PMH0016289/. Retrieved September 17, 2014.

[45] http://www.ncbi.nlm.nih.gov/pubmedhealth/PMH0004366/. Retrieved September 17, 2014.

[46] Wasmer AL. Reviewed by Geehr, EC M.D. Ending Endometriosis Pain: An Expert Q&A. *Learn About Endometriosis Symptoms and Treatments.* Special to Lifescript. Special thanks to David Redwine, MD. 2014 Jul 28. N pag. Retrieved via http://www.lifescript.com/health/centers/pms/articles/ending_endometriosis_pain_an_expert_qa.aspx. August 23, 2014.

[47] http://www.nlm.nih.gov/medlineplus/uterinefibroids.html. Retrieved September 22, 2014.

[48] http://www.mayoclinic.org/diseases-conditions/endometriosis/basics/treatment/con-20013968. Retrieved November 21, 2014.

[49] http://www.hammernutrition.com/hnt/770/. Retrieved November 15, 2014.

[50] http://www.hammernutrition.com/knowledge/electrolyte-replenishment-why-it-146-s-so-important-and-how-to-do-it-right.1274.html. Retrieved November 15, 2014.

[51] Pitchford P. Healing With Whole Foods: Asian Traditions and Modern Nutrition (3rd Edition). Paperback – November 5, 2002. ISBN-13: 9781556434303. North Atlantic Books, Berkeley, CA. Pgs 62, 621, 622.

[52] http://herbs.lovetoknow.com/Turmeric_for_Fibroids. Retrieved March 30, 2014.

[53] http://americanpregnancy.org/gettingpregnant/understandingovulation.html. Retrieved March 30, 2014.

[54] Bruner-Tran KL, Herington JL, Duleba AJ, Taylor HS, Osteen KG. Medical Management of Endometriosis: Emerging Evidence Linking Inflammation to Disease Pathophysiology. Minerva Ginecol. 2013 Apr;65(2):199-213. Retrieved via http://www.ncbi.nlm.nih.gov/pubmed/23598784. September 17, 2014.

[55] Lutgendorf SK, Kreder KJ, Rothrock NE, Hoffman A, Kirschbaum C, Sternberg EM, Zimmerman MB, Ratliff TL. Diurnal Cortisol Variations And Symptoms In Patients With Interstitial Cystitis. J Urol. 2002 Mar;167(3):1338-43. Retrieved via http://www.jurology.com/article/S0022-5347(05)65295-0/fulltext. August 23, 2014.

[56] Simon H MD, Zieve D, MD, MHA (Reviewers.) Last Reviewed on 01/30/2013. Stress. N pag. Retrieved via http://umm.edu/health/medical/reports/articles/stress#ixzz30DAG9600. September 17, 2014.

[57] Harber VJ, Sutton JR. Endorphins and Exercise. Sports Med. 1984 Mar-Apr;1(2):154-71. Retreived via www.ncbi.nlm.nih.gov. September 7, 2015.

[58] Sharma A MD, Madaan V MD, Petty F MD PhD. Exercise for Mental Health. Prim Care Companion J Clin Psychiatry. 2006; 8(2): 106. Retrieved via http://www.ncbi.nlm.gov. September 7, 2015.

[59] Taylor T, Dluhy RG, Williams GH. Beta-Endorphin Suppresses Adrenocorticotropin and Cortisol Levels in Normal Human Subjects. J Clin Endocrinol Metab. 1983 Sep;57(3):592-6. Retrieved via http://www.ncbi.nlm.nih.gov/pubmed/6308033. September 17, 2014.

Index

Anatomy of the pelvic floor	14-25, 39
Anxiety	143-149
Autonomic nervous system	20, 144, 157-158
Calcified mass	23, 229-232, 252, 259-262, 268
Childbirth	28, 53, 69, 99, 121, 185-187, 191, 200, 277, 279
Colpocele, see also Vaginocele	191-193
Communication	26, 29-30, 95, 127, 136, 193, 235, 270, 277
Core	68, 77-78, 109-110, 112-118, 120, 146-147, 159, 172-174, 179, 187, 193, 196, 234, 237-238, 261-262, 272-273, 274
Cortisol	125, 146-150, 174-175, 255-256, 258-260, 262
Cystocele	191-3
Detrusor muscle	20-21, 40-41, 43, 81, 124, 128-129, 131-134, 139, 141-142, 144-160, 163-164, 169, 175-177, 181-186, 212, 243, 268
Dyspareunia	215-219, 221-228, 269
Electrical vaginal stimulation	62-63, 84-86, 141, 163, 216-217, 227
Emotional stress	61, 218, 233, 258-269, 271
Enterocele	191-193
Estrogen	124-124, 147, 178-179, 188-189, 233, 244-245, 247
Endometriosis	24, 229-230, 233, 242, 244-249, 254-255, 259-260, 268
Fatigue with overexertion	41, 57-58, 69, 88, 98-101, 104-106, 11, 120-123, 126, 148, 164-168, 170-171, 174-176, 179, 182, 185-186, 192-193, 198, 237, 261
Fibroids	24, 230-231, 237, 244, 246, 254, 259-261
Frequency, urinary	23, 49, 60, 128-129, 135, 138-139, 141, 143-145, 152, 154-156, 158, 160, 163-163, 170-175, 179, 182, 186, 212, 216, 242-243
Hip flexor muscles	73, 77, 120-121, 171-173, 203-204, 214, 219, 222, 226, 232, 234, 246-247, 252-254, 264-266, 268, 273, 275

(See also iliacus, psoas,

and iliopsoas muscles)	
Iliacus muscle	73, 77, 120-121, 171-173, 203-204, 214,
(See also hip flexor	219, 222, 226, 232, 234, 246-247, 252-
muscles)	254, 264-266, 268, 273, 275
Iliopsoas muscle	73, 77, 120-121, 171-173, 203-204, 214,
(See also hip flexor	219, 222, 226, 232, 234, 246-247, 252-
muscles)	254, 264-266, 268, 273, 275
Incomplete void	23, 60, 156-160, 163-164, 166, 171-172, 174-175, 177-179, 186, 203, 212-214, 216, 218-219, 242
Interstitial cystitis	24, 229, 237, 242-244, 254, 256, 259-260, 262
Kegel	22, 35, 39, 41-65, 68, 80, 82, 85-110, 112-114, 183-123, 133-137, 141, 145, 149, 155, 159-160, 162, 165, 168-178, 183, 188-189, 192, 195, 198, 205-208, 215-217, 224, 226, 238, 243, 252, 261-263, 273, 276
Levator ani	4-25, 28-31, 25-229, 232-239, 242-244,
(See also pelvic floor	252-253,259, 261, 264-276
muscles)	
Masses	23, 229-233
Micturition center	39-40, 51, 131-141, 144, 148, 157, 163, 169, 175-177, 212-213, 243
Nerves, irritation	68-73
Nutrition	239-242, 244
Painful intercourse	215-219, 221-228, 269
(See also Dyspareunia)	
Pelvic asymmetry	22, 23, 68, 72, 77, 112, 114-115, 120, 176, 181,211, 213-214, 220, 234
Pelvic floor muscles	4-25, 28-31, 25-229, 232-239, 242-244, 252-253,259, 261, 264-276
(See also Levator ani and Pubococcygeus)	
Contraction of	22, 35, 39, 41-65, 68, 80, 82, 85-110,
(See also Kegel)	112-114, 183-123, 133-137, 141, 145, 149, 155, 159-160, 162, 165, 168-178, 183, 188-189, 192, 195, 198, 205-208, 215-217, 224, 226, 238, 243, 252, 261-263, 273, 276

Release of (See also lava flow)	161, 170, 177-178, 206-207, 215, 226-227, 243, 265
Pelvic pain	24, 270-271
Posture	68-73
Pregnancy	181-185
Prolapse (See also Rectocele, Cystocele, Vaginocele, Colpocele, Enterocele, Urethrocele)	24, 191-3
Prostate	272
Psoas muscle	73, 77, 120-121, 171-173, 203-204, 214, 219, 222, 226, 232, 234, 246-247, 252-254, 264-266, 268, 273, 275
Pubococcygeus muscle (See also pelvic floor muscles)	4-25, 28-31, 25-229, 232-239, 242-244, 252-253, 259, 261, 264-276
Rectocele	191-193
Scoliosis and pelvic floor dysfunction	68-73
Sling surgery	193-194
Spinal complications	68-73
Stress	143-146, 258-266
Stress urinary incontinence	81-127, 132, 134, 141
Transverse abdominis	77-78, 115-122, 173, 193, 237-238, 252, 273
Trauma (Including abuse, emotional trauma, sexual trauma)	26-29, 37-53, 200-271
Turmeric	244-245
Urgency, urinary	23, 49, 60, 128-129, 135, 138-139, 141, 143-145, 152, 154-156, 158, 160, 163-163, 170-175, 179, 182, 186, 212, 216, 242-243
Urethrocele	191-193
Urination	14, 39-41
Vaginocele (See also Colpocele)	191-193

Made in the USA
Middletown, DE
26 March 2021